PROGRESS IN METABOLIC SYNDROME RESEARCH

PROGRESS IN METABOLIC SYNDROME RESEARCH

GEORGE T. ULRIG
EDITOR

Nova Biomedical Books
New York

For permission to use material from this book please contact us:
Telephone 631-231-7269; Fax 631-231-8175
Web Site: http://www.novapublishers.com

NOTICE TO THE READER

The Publisher has taken reasonable care in the preparation of this book, but makes no expressed or implied warranty of any kind and assumes no responsibility for any errors or omissions. No liability is assumed for incidental or consequential damages in connection with or arising out of information contained in this book. The Publisher shall not be liable for any special, consequential, or exemplary damages resulting, in whole or in part, from the readers' use of, or reliance upon, this material.

Independent verification should be sought for any data, advice or recommendations contained in this book. In addition, no responsibility is assumed by the publisher for any injury and/or damage to persons or property arising from any methods, products, instructions, ideas or otherwise contained in this publication.

This publication is designed to provide accurate and authoritative information with regard to the subject matter cover herein. It is sold with the clear understanding that the Publisher is not engaged in rendering legal or any other professional services. If legal, medical or any other expert assistance is required, the services of a competent person should be sought. FROM A DECLARATION OF PARTICIPANTS JOINTLY ADOPTED BY A COMMITTEE OF THE AMERICAN BAR ASSOCIATION AND A COMMITTEE OF PUBLISHERS.

Library of Congress Cataloging-in-Publication Data

Progress in metabolic syndrome research / William H. Dunleavy, (editor).
　　p. ; cm.
Includes bibliographical references and index.
ISBN 1-60021-179-8
1. Metabolic syndrome--Research. 2. Coronary heart disease--Prevention--Research. 3. Lipids--Metabolism--Disorders--Research. I. Dunleavy, William H.
[DNLM: 1. Metabolic Syndrome X--etiology. 2. Diabetes Mellitus, Type 2--prevention & control. 3. Polymorphism, Genetic.　WK 820 P9645 2006]
RC662.4.P76　　　　　　　　　　　　　　　　　　　　　　　　　　　　2006
616.1'23050072--dc22　　　　　　　　　　　　　　　　　　　　　2006012507

Published by Nova Science Publishers, Inc. ✤*New York*

Contents

Preface

In chapter I, small, dense LDL are associated with increased risk for cardiovascular disease and diabetes mellitus and a reduction in LDL size has been reported in patients with acute myocardial infarction, angina pectoris or in patients with non-coronary forms of atherosclerosis. LDL size has been accepted as an important predictor of cardiovascular events and progression of coronary artery disease as well as an emerging cardiovascular risk factor by the National Cholesterol Education Program Adult Treatment Panel III. Importantly, small, dense LDL, with elevated triglyceride levels and low HDL-cholesterol concentrations, constitute the "atherogenic lipoprotein phenotype", a form of atherogenic dyslipidemia that is a feature of type 2 diabetes and the metabolic syndrome. LDL size and subclasses show specific alterations in patients with the metabolic syndrome that probably significantly increase their cardiovascular risk; however, so far it has not been recommended by the international scientific societies to incorporate LDL size measurements in treatment plans, when hypolipidemic therapies are installed. It is very well known that patients with type 2 diabetes are at very high cardiovascular risk and it is still on debate if the treatment goals may be identical or whether there are distinct groups with different cardiovascular risk and hence different treatment goals. Measurements beyond traditional lipids, such as on the presence of small, dense LDL in patients with the metabolic syndrome, may help to identify cardiovascular risk subgroups. In addition, it might be possible in the future to individualize hypolipidemic treatments if more than the traditional lipids are taken into account. Particularly LDL size measurements may help to assess cardiovascular risk within the metabolic syndrome and adapt the treatment goals thereafter.

Chapter II informs about, insulin is an essential hormone with important roles in glucose homeostasis and anabolic metabolism. Cellular and/or molecular defects in insulin action result in a state of *insulin resistance*, which is an essential feature of the diseases type 2 diabetes and the metabolic syndrome. One of the largest correlations to insulin resistance is obesity; specifically the enlargement of adipose tissue in the abdomen. This correlation is unmistakably obvious today as the twin epidemics of obesity and type 2 diabetes have co-emerged. One of the biggest challenges in the field of diabetes research is to determine how the increase in visceral adiposity leads to impaired insulin action. Recently, two hypothetical mechanisms have transpired: (a) obesity shifts the secretory profile of adipose tissue to favor a reduction in nutrient uptake by creating insulin resistance, and/or (b) overloaded fat cells and the increased caloric intake common in obesity leads to the inappropriate storage of lipids in non-adipose tissues where they antagonize insulin action. This review summarizes recent findings implicating each mechanism, alone or in concert, in the etiology of obesity-induced insulin resistance.

Chapter III presents, type 2 diabetes (type 2 DM) is strongly associated with obesity. The obesity epidemic has been accompanied during the last decade by a 25% increase in the prevalence of type 2 DM.

Diabetes confers an increased risk of cardiovascular disease, kidney disease and microvascular complications including nephropathy, retinopathy and neuropathy. Glycemic and blood pressure control were both shown to decrease microvascular and macrovascular risk in patients with but it was not until recently that it was shown that can be prevented, or at least delayed by lifestyle changes and pharmacologic therapy.

Lifestyle changes, including weight reduction, an increase in fiber consumption among other nutritional changes, and an increase in physical activity, was shown to be highly effective in preventing type 2 DM in high risk patients with impaired glucose tolerance. In the Diabetes Prevention Program Study, patients randomized to lifestyle changes had a 58% reduced risk for developing diabetes, compared to the control group, while patients treated with metformin had a 31% risk reduction. Pharmacotherapy, specifically metformin, was also shown to be effective in the prevention of type 2 DM, although less so than lifestyle changes. Patients treated with orlistat, a lipase inhibitor, and lifestyle changes had a 37% risk reduction for developing diabetes, while patients treated with acarbose (an α-glusidase inhibitor), had a 25% risk reduction.

The diabetes epidemic poses a worldwide health challenge due to its severe health consequences. Presently, several drugs has been shown to effective in preventing type 2 DM and many others are now being evaluated for this role. Lifestyle changes have been shown to be the most effective diabetes prevention strategy, particularly in patients with IGT, and should be widely implemented as primary therapy.

In chapter IV, the metabolic syndrome consists of a constellation of risk factors including obesity, glucose intolerance, hypertension, and dyslipidemia in the setting of insulin resistance that confers an increased risk of cardiovascular disease and type 2 diabetes. Although the major pathophysiologic mechanisms are still in the process of being elucidated, the possible role of inflammation, cytokines, and atherogenic markers has received attention lately. Recent studies suggest that inflammatory markers like C-reactive protein (CRP), Interleukin (IL)-6, and Tumor Necrosis Factor (TNF)-α mirror oxidative stress and may be instrumental in the final pathway of adverse vascular outcomes in the metabolic syndrome. Other adipocytokines produced by fatty tissue are also altered, with lower levels of adiponectin and increased leptin and resistin. Elevated Plasminogen Activator Inhibitor (PAI)-1 and fibrinogen levels, and derangement in clotting factors correlate with the degree of insulin resistance and may contribute to the prothrombotic tendency. Taken together, these abnormalities shift the balance of endothelial function towards an abnormal state that heightens the risk of atherothrombosis. Lifestyle factors and medications can have a profound effect in modifying these parameters. The phenomenal increase in the prevalence of obesity has accentuated the various clinical manifestations and pathopysiologic underpinnings of this epidemic. Continued research looking at the role of inflammation and cytokines in the genesis and propagation of the metabolic syndrome should provide a window into its pathogenesis at the cellular and humoral level, improve the understanding of disease mechanisms, and open up possibilities for effective therapeutic interventions in the future.

Chapter V reviews Metabolic syndrome (MS) comprises a range of alterations associated with glucose and lipid homeostasis disturbances, all conditions which are strongly influenced by each individual's genetic and environmental factors. In addition to Insulin resistance, abdominal obesity and dyslipidemia, arterial blood pressure, pro-inflammatory and pro-thrombotic states have also been included as major components of MS. This multifaceted composition implies that many metabolic pathways could be genetically altered. In humans, there has been described a number of single nucleotide polymorphisms (SNP) and deletion/insertion polymorphisms in different genes linked to glucose metabolism (Insulin receptor *IR*, protein tyrosine phosphatase 1β PTPβ), blood pressure (beta-adrenergic receptors *BAR*, renin-angiotensin system RAS, Nitric Oxide Sintase NOS), lipoprotein variations (Cholesteryl ester transfer protein *CETP*, Apolipoproteins AI, C-III, and E), lower Body Mass Index (Leptin, Peroxisome proliferator-activated receptors *PPAR*, uncoupling protein *UCP*), some inflammatory components (C Reactive protein *CRP*) and the hemostatic system (plasminogen-activator inhibitor *PAI-1*), among others. The purpose of this review is to compile recent evidence that could link genetic variations of different genes with the phenotypic features of MS.

In: Progress in Metabolic Syndrome Research
Editor: G.T. Ulrig, pp. 1-37

ISBN 1-60021-179-8
© 2006 Nova Science Publishers, Inc.

Chapter I

Low-Density-Lipoproteins Heterogeneity and the Metabolic Syndrome

Manfredi Rizzo[1], and Kaspar Berneis[2]*
[1]Department of Clinical Medicine and Emerging Diseases,
University of Palermo, Italy;
[2]Division of Endocrinology and Diabetology,
University Hospital Zurich, Switzerland.

Abstract

Small, dense LDL are associated with increased risk for cardiovascular disease and diabetes mellitus and a reduction in LDL size has been reported in patients with acute myocardial infarction, angina pectoris or in patients with non-coronary forms of atherosclerosis. LDL size has been accepted as an important predictor of cardiovascular events and progression of coronary artery disease as well as an emerging cardiovascular risk factor by the National Cholesterol Education Program Adult Treatment Panel III. Importantly, small, dense LDL, with elevated triglyceride levels and low HDL-cholesterol concentrations, constitute the "atherogenic lipoprotein phenotype", a form of atherogenic dyslipidemia that is a feature of type 2 diabetes and the metabolic syndrome. LDL size and subclasses show specific alterations in patients with the metabolic syndrome that probably significantly increase their cardiovascular risk; however, so far it has not been recommended by the international scientific societies to incorporate LDL size measurements in treatment plans, when hypolipidemic therapies are installed. It is very well known that patients with type 2 diabetes are at very high cardiovascular risk and it is still on debate if the treatment goals may be identical or whether there are

---

* Correspondence concerning this article should be addressed to Dr. Manfredi Rizzo, Dipartimento di Medicina Clinica e delle Patologie Emergenti, Universita' di Palermo, Via del Vespro, 141, 90127 – Palermo – Italy. Ph. +39 (091) 6552945; Fax: +39 (091) 6552982. E-mail: mrizzo@unipa.it.

distinct groups with different cardiovascular risk and hence different treatment goals. Measurements beyond traditional lipids, such as on the presence of small, dense LDL in patients with the metabolic syndrome, may help to identify cardiovascular risk subgroups. In addition, it might be possible in the future to individualize hypolipidemic treatments if more than the traditional lipids are taken into account. Particularly LDL size measurements may help to assess cardiovascular risk within the metabolic syndrome and adapt the treatment goals thereafter.

Keywords: Small, dense LDL; Coronary heart disease; Atherosclerosis; Prevention; Metabolic syndrome.

Introduction

Several expert groups have suggested in the past years diagnostic criteria to be used in clinical practice to identify patients with metabolic syndrome, and these definitions have been somewhat different [1-8]. As recently stated by the joint American Heart Association/National Heart, Lung, and Blood Institute Scientific Statement on "Diagnosis and Management of the Metabolic Syndrome" III [8], all the proposed classifications have in common the concept that the metabolic syndrome represent a constellation of interrelated risk factors of metabolic origin ("metabolic risk factors") that appear to directly promote the development of atherosclerotic cardiovascular disease. The metabolic risk factors include elevated blood pressure, elevated plasma glucose and atherogenic dyslipidemia, which consists of an aggregation of lipoprotein abnormalities including elevated plasma triglyceride levels, increased small, dense low-density-lipoproteins (LDL), and reduced high-density-lipoproteins (HDL)-cholesterol concentrations.

This form of dyslipidemia, also known as "atherogenic lipoprotein phenotype" or "lipid triad" represents a partially heritable trait and is associated with increased cardiovascular risk [9-11]. It has also been suggested that the clinical importance of the atherogenic lipoprotein phenotype probably exceeds that of LDL-cholesterol, because many more patients with coronary artery disease are found to have this trait compared to those with hypercholesterolaemia [12,13]. LDL size in humans does not show a normal, but a bimodal distribution and can be separated into two phenotypes, "pattern A" when larger, more buoyant LDL and "pattern B" when smaller, more dense LDL predominate [14-17]. Small, dense LDL are associated with the metabolic syndrome and with increased risk for cardiovascular disease and diabetes mellitus [16-18]. LDL size seems also to be an important predictor of cardiovascular events and progression of coronary artery disease (CAD) [18,19]. In addition, the predominance of small dense LDL has been accepted as an emerging cardiovascular risk factor by the National Cholesterol Education Program Adult Treatment Panel III [3].

Heterogeneity of LDL Particles

LDL comprise multiple distinct subclasses that differ in size, density, physicochemical composition, metabolic behaviour and atherogenicity. There are at least four major subspecies of LDL: large LDL-I, medium LDL-II, small LDL-III, very small LDL-IV [16,20] (Figure 1). LDL subclasses show differences in the surface lipid content and certain features of the apolipoprotein B100 structure probably contribute to size changes of these particles. Based on measurement of peak particle diameter or ultracentrifugal density, individuals generally cluster into two broad subgroups, the majority with a predominance of larger or medium sized LDL (LDL pattern A) and a substantial minority with a higher proportion of smaller LDL particles (LDL pattern B) [10,16-19].

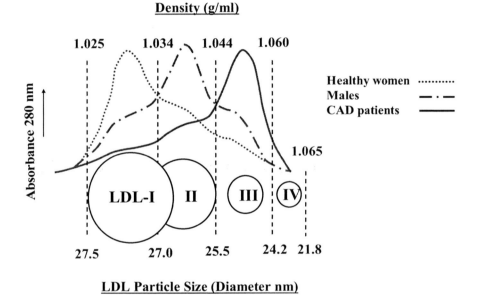

Figure 1. LDL subclass distribution according to size and density (as modified from 34,38). CAD: coronary artery disease.

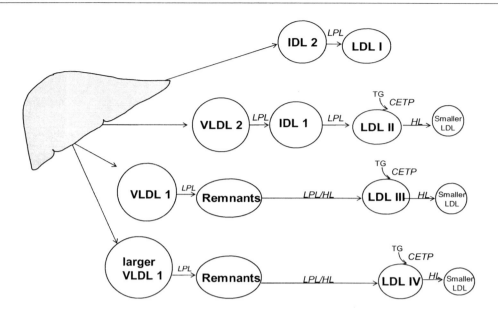

Figure 2. Hypothetical metabolic scheme incorporating proposed pathways for the production of the major LDL subclasses (as modified from 16). VLDL: very low density lipoproteins; IDL: intermediate density lipoproteins; TG: triglycerides; LPL: lipoprotein lipase; HL: hepatic lipase; CETP: cholesterol ester transfer protein.

It has been suggested that there are parallel metabolic channels within the delipidation cascade from very low-density-lipoproteins (VLDL) to LDL [16] (Figure 2). A metabolic relationship between large VLDL particles and small LDL particles has been demonstrated using stable isotopes in subjects with a predominance of small dense LDL [21]. Kinetic analysis of tracer studies in humans demonstrate that LDL particles show an initial rapid plasma decay which is due to both intra-extravascular exchange and catabolism of LDL These studies have not yet identified the specific precursors of individual LDL subclasses, however there are data from animal models suggesting that separate pathways may be responsible for the generation of distinct LDL particles [16,22]. Inverse correlation's of changes in large LDL (LDL-I) and small LDL (LDL-III) and of changes of medium sized LDL (LDL II) and very small LDL (LDL IV) in dietary intervention studies raise the possibility of precursor-product relationships between distinct LDL subclasses [16] (Figure 3).

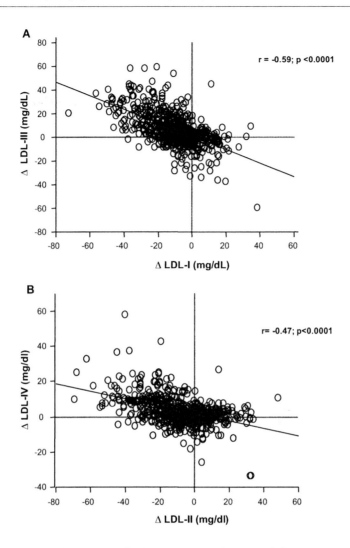

Figure 3. Reciprocal relationships between diet induced changes in LDL subclasses as measured by analytical ultracentrifugation (as modified from 16).

Activity of lipolytic enzymes is related to the size of LDL particles. A significant inverse relationship between postheparin lipoprotein lipase (LpL) activity and small dense LDL has been demonstrated and increases of LpL by high fat diet was associated with an increase of large LDL and decrease of small dense LDL. Reduced activity of LpL and increased activity of hepatic lipase has been shown in subjects with the pattern B phenotype [22]. Hepatic lipase (HL) has a higher affinity for LDL than LpL and is positively correlated with plasma triglycerides, apolipoprotein B, mass of large VLDL and small dense LDL, but not with the mass of large LDL, suggesting an important role for HL in the lipolytic conversion of these particles [22]. The strong relationship of LDL size and triglycerides (Figure 4) is based on their importance as substrates for the size reduction of LDL particles: by exchange of cholesteryl esters with triglycerides, LDL can become triglyceride-enriched and can be further processed by lipases.

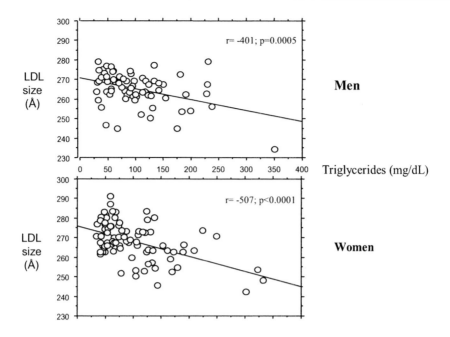

Figure 4. Spearman correlations between plasma triglyeride levels and LDL peak particle size in men and women from Ustica, a mediterranean island (as modified from 24).

LDL Subclass Phenotype Assignment

Particle size distribution of plasma LDL subfractions can be measured by different laboratory techniques, including analytical, preparative and nonequilibrium density gradient ultracentrifugation, as well as nuclear magnetic resonance [23]. However, the most common procedure is represented by the 2-16% gradient gel electrophoresis at 10°C using a Tris (0.09 M)- boric acid (0.08 M)- Na_2 EDTA(0.003 M) buffer (pH 8.3) [18,19]. In details, plasma is adjusted to 20% sucrose, and 3 to 10 µL are applied to the gel. Potentials are set at 40 mV (15 minutes), 80 mV (15 minutes), and 125 mV (24 hours). Gels are fixed and stained for lipids in a solution containing oil red O in 60% ethanol at 55°C, for proteins in a solution containing 0.1% Coomassie brilliant blue R-250, 50% ethanol and 9% acetic acid and then scanned with a densitometer. Molecular diameters are determined on the basis of migration distance by comparison with standards of known diameter [18,19].

Assignment of LDL subclass phenotypes is based on particle diameter of the major plasma LDL peak: LDL pattern A (larger, more buoyant LDL) is defined as an LDL subclass pattern with the major gradient gel peak at a particle diameter of 258 Å or greater, whereas the major peak of LDL pattern B (small, dense LDL) is at a particle diameter of less than 258 Å [18,19].

It has been shown that LDL phenotype is genetically influenced with a heritability ranging from 35-45% and the predominance of small dense LDL is commonly found in conjunction with familial disorders of lipoprotein metabolism that are associated with increased risk of premature coronary artery disease [16]. The prevalence of the pattern B phenotype is approximately 30% in adult men, 5-10% in young men and women < 20yrs and approximately 15-25% in postmenopausal women, but a number of non-genetic (environmental) factors may influence the expression of this phenotype, including abdominal adiposity, oral contraceptive use and dietary factors [24].

Atherogenicity of Small, Dense LDL

Several reasons have been suggested for atherogenicity of small dense LDL. Smaller, denser LDL are taken up more easily by arterial tissue than larger LDL [25], suggesting greater transendothelial transport of smaller particles. In addition, smaller LDL particles may also have decreased receptor-mediated uptake and increased proteoglycan binding [26]. Sialic acid, perhaps because of its exposure at the LDL surface, plays a determinant role in the in vitro association of LDL with the polyanionic proteoglycans [27] and it has been shown that sialic acid content of LDL particles of subjects with the pattern B phenotype is reduced.

Further, it has been shown that oxidative susceptibility increases and antioxidant concentrations decreases with decreasing LDL size [28]. Altered properties of the surface lipid layer associated with reduced content of free cholesterol [29] and increased content of polyunsaturated fatty acids [30] might contribute to enhanced oxidative susceptibility of small dense LDL.

Recently [31] we have chosen the model of apoB transgenic mice to evaluate the kinetic behaviour of human LDL particles of different size in vivo in a genetically homogeneous recipient avoiding other metabolic differences that could influence LDL metabolism. We found that small LDL particles have intrinsic features that lead to retarded metabolism and decreased intra-extravascular equilibration compared to medium sized LDL: these properties may contribute to greater atherogenicity of small dense LDL.

Small, Dense LDL and Cardiovascular Risk

To date, the magnitude and independence of the association of LDL size with cardiovascular diseases has been tested in many studies, including cross-sectional and prospective epidemiologic as well as clinical intervention trials [32-82]. The vast majority, but not all, of these trials demonstrate a significant univariate association of small, dense LDL with increased CHD risk. However, LDL size is rarely a significant and independent predictor of CHD risk after multivariate adjustment for confounding variables, in particular plasma triglyceride levels and HDL-cholesterol concentrations (Table 1).

Table 1. Univariate and multivariate analyses on the association of small, dense LDL particle size with cardiovascular diseases. CS: cross-sectional; P: prospective (as modified from 18)

Author	Study design	Uni-variate	Multi-variate	Author	Study design	Uni-variate	Multi-variate
Crouse 32	CS	Yes	No	Skoglund 57	CS	Yes	Yes
Austin 33	CS	Yes	No	Zambon 58	P	Yes	Yes
Griffin 34	CS	Yes	No	Austin 59	P	Yes	No
Tornvall 35	CS	Yes	---	Hulthe 60	CS	No	---
Campos 36	CS	Yes	No	Hulthe 61	CS	Yes	---
Coresh 37	CS	Yes	No	Bokemark 62	CS	Yes	No
Griffin 38	CS	Yes	Yes	Campos 63	P	No	No
Campos 39	CS	No	No	Kamigaki 64	CS	Yes	No
Sherrard 40	CS	No	---	Rosenson 65	P	Yes	Yes
Rajman 41	CS	No	---	Blake 66	P	Yes	No
Stampfer 42	P	Yes	No	Kuller 67	P	Yes	No
Gardner 43	P	Yes	Yes	Liu 68	CS	Yes	Yes
Miller 44	P	Yes	No	Koba 69	CS	Yes	Yes
Mack 45	P	Yes	No	Vakkilainen 70	P	Yes	No
Lamarche 46	P	Yes	Yes	Slowik 71	CS	Yes	---
Gray 47	CS	No	---	Hallman 72	CS	Yes	---
Wahi 48	CS	No	---	Watanabe 73	CS	Yes	---
Slyper 49	CS	No	---	Wallenfeldt 74	P	Yes	---
Freedman 50	CS	Yes	No	Kullo 75	CS	Yes	No
Ruotolo 51	P	Yes	No	van Tits 76	P	Yes	---
O'Neal 52	CS	Yes	Yes	Inukai 77	CS	Yes	Yes
Landray 53	CS	Yes	No	Mohan 78	CS	Yes	---
Hulthe 54	CS	Yes	---	Yoon 79	CS	Yes	Yes
Mykkanen 55	P	No	No	St. Pierre 80	P	Yes	---
Erbey 56	CS	Yes	No	Berneis 81	CS	Yes	Yes

Therefore, it cannot be excluded that the increased risk associated with smaller LDL size in univariate analyses may be a consequence of the broader pathophysiology of which small, dense LDL is a part (e.g., high triglycerides, low HDL-cholesterol, increased LDL particle number, obesity, insulin resistance, diabetes, metabolic syndrome) rather than a reflection of an intrinsic increased atherogenic potential and a clear causal relationship between small dense LDL and increased cardiovascular risk based on the present knowledge cannot be proven.

This is further complicated by the fact that at the same level of LDL-cholesterol, higher-risk pattern B individuals have significantly more particles than those with larger LDL pattern A. The number of LDL particles in plasma is conceptually very important because the arterial walls are exposed to these particles and an increased number may increase the atherogenicity independently of particle size [83]. Is the higher risk of pattern B individuals attributable to the fact that they have more LDL particles in total, or does the "quality" of smaller size contribute independently to greater CHD risk?

Assessment of LDL particle size by gradient gel electrophoresis does not provide information about the concentration or number of small, dense LDL particles, which has been historically estimated by measuring apo B concentrations [84]. Rader [85] and Sniderman [86] reviewed thirty-two trials that studied the relationship of plasma apo B concentrations and CHD risk, but data supporting a superior association of apo B versus other lipid parameters were not consistent.

LDL particle number is currently assessed by nuclear magnetic resonance, which provides data on both LDL particle size and concentration [87]. Higher LDL particle concentrations seem to be very important in determining CHD risk [88,89]; however, few studies have assessed if the quantity rather than the quality of small, dense LDL may be stronger associated with CHD risk [65-67,82]. In these studies the number of total and smaller LDL particles has consistently been shown to be a significant and independent predictor of CHD risk following multivariate adjustment for lipid variables [65-67, 82].

In addition, studies in which not only the LDL-cholesterol concentration and particle size were measured, but also LDL particle numbers in plasma, have provided important information on the risk of CHD [83,87]. It is notable that when both number of LDL particles and LDL size are measured in the same study population, small, dense LDL particles are frequently not significantly associated with CHD risk [44,46,51,66,67]. In summary, all these data underline the clinical importance of assessing LDL particle number in order to adequately establish the risk of CHD associated with the presence of small, dense LDL particles [84,87].

Small, Dense LDL and Cardiovascular Diseases

Small, Dense LDL and Acute Myocardial Infarction

Acute myocardial infarction and the atherogenic lipoprotein phenotype seem to share a similar array of interrelated metabolic aberrations, including modifications in plasma lipids and lipoproteins as well as a relative resistance to insulin-mediated glucose uptake. The common lipid alterations observed during the acute phase of myocardial infarction include a rise of triglyceride levels and a fall of total, LDL- and HDL-cholesterol concentrations [90-92] and such modifications have a great clinical relevance since they must be taken into account in making therapeutic decisions [93].

However, despite a number of data regarding the modifications of total plasma lipoprotein fractions during a myocardial infarction, it is less defined whether or not also the LDL peak particle size is modified by the acute phase and therefore the best time to measure it. We recently found [94] in a group of subjects admitted to hospital for a myocardial infarction, and followed until the discharge and three months after the event, that the reduction of LDL peak particle size is premature and persist during the hospitalisation, with a significant increase three months after the myocardial infarction. In addition, the timing of these changes seemed to precede those of all other lipoproteins.

Notably, it has been recently shown that even angina itself (on the background of coronary artery spasm), without atherosclerosis, may lower LDL size [95].

Small, Dense LDL and Carotid Artery Disease

Landray et al. in 1998 [53] first showed an association between small, dense LDL and asymptomatic carotid atherosclerosis. This preliminary finding was confirmed by other similar studies in healthy individuals [57,62,72]. In addition, LDL size was significantly correlated (inversely) with carotid intima media thickness (IMT) in asymptomatic members of familial combined hyperlipidemia families [68], in subjects with familial hypercholesterolemia [76] and in patients with vascular dementia or Alzheimer's disease [73]. By contrast, no association between LDL size and IMT was found in adults with growth hormone deficiency [96] or familial hypercholesterolemia [97].

Hulthe et al. found a significant relationship between LDL size and the occurrence of preclinical and clinical carotid atherosclerosis [54,61]; however, the authors did not find any association when they studied patients with hypercholesterolemia [60]. In addition, we recently demonstrated [81] that LDL size is significantly associated with carotid IMT in patients with type 2 diabetes and multivariate analysis revealed that LDL size was the strongest predictor of IMT within all lipid parameters and the second strongest predictor (after smoking) among all traditional cardiovascular risk factors (Table 2).

Table 2. LDL subclass particle concentrations (mean±SD, in nmol/l) by nuclear magnetic resonance in insulin-sensitive (IS), insulin-resistant (IR), and type 2 diabetic (DM) subjects (as modified from 88)

	IS	IR	DM	IR vs IS	DM vs IS
				p=	p=
Large	589 ± 325	534 ± 357	385 ± 418	0.4457	**0.0058**
Intermediate	238 ± 316	213 ± 271	385 ± 425	0.7218	**0.0312**
Small	366 ± 398	668 ± 599	805 ± 712	**0.0088**	**0.0002**

Regarding clinical trials, Van Tits et al. [76] showed an association between IMT regression and baseline LDL size (under statin therapy with atorvastatin and simvastatin) and this was confirmed by Wallenfeldt et al. [74] in a 3 years follow-up of 313 58-years-old subjects. These findings are consistent with a role of LDL size in modulating carotid atherosclerosis regression.

Small, Dense LDL and Peripheral Arterial Disease

The association between PAD and plasma lipids and lipoproteins has not been as extensively investigated as for coronary artery disease and results have been less conclusive so far. However, many studies have showed that PAD is associated with elevated plasma total cholesterol or triglyceride levels and with reduced plasma HDL-cholesterol concentrations (as reviewed in 52).

In fact, to-date only two published studies have directly examined the association of LDL size with the presence of PAD [52,98], with contrasting results. Lupattelli et al [98] didn't find any difference in the LDL size between a group of 16 male normolipemic non-diabetic PAD patients and a group of 16 health control subjects matched for gender, age and body mass index. O'Neal et al [52] have performed a similar study but on a larger number of patients and they found that a smaller LDL particle size was associated with the presence of PAD in absence or presence of diabetes.

Due to the lack in literature, we recently measured the LDL peak particle size in a group of 50 adult males with PAD (Rizzo M. and Berneis K., unpublished data) in order to assess the prevalence of LDL phenotype pattern B and to evaluate if LDL size may be a predictor of future cardiovascular events in this category of patients and preliminary findings are available for the baseline evaluation. We found an elevated prevalence of LDL phenotype pattern B in patients with PAD (32%), a value that is much higher than what we previously found in healthy adult males in our area (16%) [24] and that is similar to what we found in our patients with acute myocardial infarction (30%) [94].

It has been recently stated by the National Cholesterol Education Program Adult Treatment Panel III that clinical forms of non-coronary atherosclerosis carry a risk for coronary heart disease (CHD) equal to those with established CHD [3]. These conditions include peripheral arterial disease, symptomatic (transient ischemic attack or stroke of carotid origin) and asymptomatic (>50% stenosis on angiography or ultrasound) carotid artery disease and abdominal aortic aneurysm [3]. Therefore, our findings may support the usefulness to extend LDL size measurement as much as possible to patients with PAD, for a better management of their secondary cardiovascular prevention.

Small, Dense LDL and Abdominal Aortic Aneurysms

To our knowledge, no published studies directly examined the LDL size in patients with abdominal aortic aneurysm (AAA). Gorter et al. [99] recently found an elevated prevalence of the metabolic syndrome (as defined by the National Cholesterol Education Program ATP III) in patients with manifest atherosclerotic vascular disease, including patients with AAA. The Adult Treatment Panel III guidelines [3] define the metabolic syndrome as the concomitant presence of at least three components within: abdominal obesity, low plasma HDL-cholesterol levels, elevated plasma tryglicerides concentrations, high fasting glucose levels and elevated blood pressure.

Since these clinical characteristics are common features of patients with the predominance of small, dense LDL [11], it is likely that the presence of AAA may be associated with reduced LDL size. Due to the lack in literature, we recently examined the LDL peak particle size in a group of 22 male adult patients with AAA compared to 22 healthy subjects matched for gender and age, used as controls (Rizzo M. and Berneis K., unpublished data). We found that patients with AAA had a significantly smaller LDL size and a different LDL subclass distribution, with lower levels of the smallest LDL (LDL-I) and increased levels of intermediate-size particles (LDL-II A and LDL-II B).

Small, Dense LDL and Diabetes

Hypertriglyceridemia, low HDL cholesterol and an increased fraction of small dense LDL particles characterise diabetic dyslipidemia [100-102], while LDL or total cholesterol are generally not increased in diabetes patients except for a slight increase of LDL cholesterol in women [103]. In addition, small dense LDL is associated with the cluster of risk factors that characterise the insulin resistance syndrome [104].

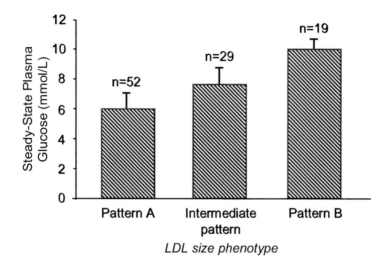

Figure 5. LDL phenotypes in patients with insulin resistance (as modified from 106).

Interestingly, subjects with predominance of small dense LDL have a greater than two fold increased risk for developing type 2 diabetes mellitus, independent from age, sex, glucose tolerance and body mass index. An increase of peak LDL size was associated with a 16% decrease in the risk of developing type 2 diabetes mellitus [105]. It has also been shown that patients with the insulin resistance syndrome have an elevated prevalence of the LDL "pattern B" phenotype [106] (Figure 5) and this has been confirmed for diabetes, in both men and women [101,107] (Figure 6). In addition, using a euglycemic clamp technique to categorise individuals as insulin-sensitive, insulin-resistant, or type 2 diabetic, more severe states of insulin resistance were associated with smaller LDL particle size (Table 3)

Recently, we investigated the clinical significance of LDL size and LDL subclasses in diabetes type 2 patients [81]. Diabetes patients with manifest CHD had decreased LDL particle sizes and altered LDL subclass distributions, i.e. specifically more LDL III B and less LDL I and LDL II as compared to diabetes patients without established CHD. Multivariate analysis revealed that LDL size was the strongest marker of CHD as compared to nine other established cardiovascular risk factors, including plasma lipids and lipoproteins.

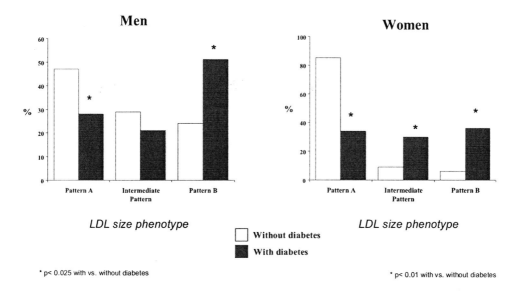

Figure 6. LDL phenotypes in men and women with diabetes (as modified from 101,107).

Table 3. Multivariate analysis of variance of 10 cardiovascular risk factors for coronary heart disease (CHD) and intima media thickness (IMT) (as modified from 81)

	Presence of IMT (MANOVA, p=)	Presence of CHD (MANOVA, p=)
Smoking (pack-years)	0.003	0.005
LDL size (angstrom)	0.03	0.002
LDL-cholesterol (mmol/L)	0.06	0.01
HDL-cholesterol (mmol/L)	0.06	0.01
Lipoprotein (a) (g/L)	0.06	0.5
Age (years)	0.2	0.9
Haemoglobin A1c (%)	0.3	0.5
C-reactive protein (mg/dL)	0.3	0.9
Systolic blood pressure (mm Hg)	0.6	0.2
Body Mass Index	0.8	0.2

Increased IMT thickness is considered a reliable surrogate marker of early atherosclerosis and it has been shown to correlate significantly with the presence of CHD and to predict coronary events [108-111]. In addition, significant relationships of IMT with other lipid parameters as LDL cholesterol [112] and apoB [113] have been demonstrated. In our study described above [81], LDL size was significantly associated with carotid IMT in diabetes type 2 patients and LDL size was the second strongest predictor of IMT, after smoking when compared to nine other cardiovascular risk factors and the strongest of all lipid parameters (Table 2).

In summary, LDL size seems to represent a marker of clinical apparent (CHD) and non-apparent (IMT) atherosclerosis in diabetes type 2. However the potential clinical value in this population that is at high risk of cardiovascular events [114] needs to be shown in prospective studies, before routine laboratory measurements of LDL size can be recommended.

Small, Dense LDL and Polycystic Ovary Syndrome

Women's health is about the prevention, screening, diagnosis, and treatment of disorders that are unique to women. Polycystic ovary syndrome (PCOS) is extremely prevalent and probably constitutes the most frequently encountered endocrinopathy in women, affecting up to 10% of women in reproductive age [115,116]

However classification criteria were always on debate. During the last two decades, the criteria for making the diagnosis of hyperandrogenic syndromes have changed several times and it has influenced the classification and the relative prevalence of the different androgen excess disorders. More recently, a meeting of experts has suggested new criteria for making diagnosis of PCOS [117]. With these new criteria, the diagnosis of PCOS can be made in patients having two of these three elements: clinical or biologic hyperandrogenism, chronic anovulation, polycystic ovaries [118].

Although PCOS is known to be associated with reproductive morbidity and increased risk for endometrial cancer, diagnosis is especially important because PCOS is now thought to increase metabolic and cardiovascular risk [115,116]. Many women with PCOS are very similar to those with the metabolic syndrome and the presence of PCOS have been accepted by the NECP as a feature of such syndrome [3,8].

Nearly 40% of women with PCOS will have impaired glucose tolerance or overt type 2 diabetes, a finding that is consistently seen across several geographic areas and ethnic groups. Moreover, women with PCOS are more likely than normally cycling women to have insulin resistance, central adiposity, dyslipidemia, and hypertension. Other markers of cardiovascular disease, such as C-reactive protein and homocysteine, have also been found to be elevated in women with PCOS [119]. In addition to serum markers, several measures of subclinical atherosclerosis, including carotid intima-media thickness and coronary artery calcium are elevated in patients with PCOS. The risk of coronary artery disease and myocardial infarction has been reported to be increased in patients with PCOS compared with regularly cycling women even if mortality because of circulatory disease may be not increased [119].

Regarding the lipid abnormalities usually seen in women with PCOS, they include low HDL-cholesterol levels and elevated triglyceride concentrations [115,116,119]. Only few authors investigated so far if such lipid alterations may be accompanied by modifications in LDL size or subclasses [120-123], but with unclear results. In order to investigate this field, we recently examined LDL size and subclasses in a group of 14 female young adult patients with PCOS compared to 14 healthy subjects matched for age and body mass index, used as controls (Berneis K., Rizzo M. and Carmina E., unpublished data). We found that patients with PCOS patients had a significantly smaller LDL size and a different LDL subclass distribution (Figure 7), with lower levels of the largest particles (LDL-I and LDL-IIA) and higher concentrations of all other smaller subspecies (LDL-II B, -IIIA, -IIIB, -IVA and -IVB).

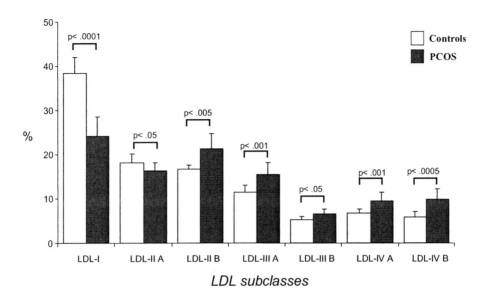

Figure 7. LDL subclasses in patients with polycystic ovary syndrome.

Small, Dense LDL and the Metabolic Syndrome

Small, dense LDL represent (with low HDL-cholesterol and elevated trygliceride concentrations) one of the three components of atherogenic dyslipidemia, that is strongly associated with the metabolic syndrome [3,8]; however, scientific guidelines support so far recommendations to manage HDL-cholesterol and trygliceride levels only [3,8].

Beyond this lipoprotein profile, small, dense LDL may be independently associated with the metabolic syndrome, but further studies are need in the future. Hulthe et al. [61] assessed the prevalence of metabolic syndrome in a population-based sample of clinically 58 years old healthy men, using the WHO definition [1]. The authors found that LDL size was significantly smaller in subjects with the metabolic syndrome, in relation to those without it (Figure 8). In addition they found that subjects with pattern B had significantly higher mean values for body mass index, blood pressures, heart rate, serum cholesterol, triglyceride levels, and plasma insulin and lower HDL levels compared with subjects with pattern A. Subjects with pattern B also had a higher prevalence of moderate to large plaques in the carotid artery compared with subjects with pattern A. Interestingly, decreasing LDL peak particle size was significantly associated with increasing IMT of the common carotid artery, the carotid artery bulb, and the common femoral artery. There was a statistically significant association between plaque occurrence and size and the LDL peak particle diameter in both the carotid and femoral arteries.

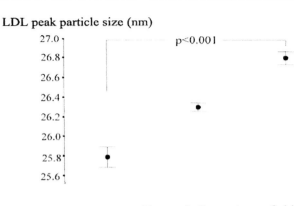

Figure 8. LDL size in patients with the metabolic syndrome (as modified from 61).

However, Haffner et al. have already shown in 1995 that LDL size is decreased in subjects with multiple metabolic disorders. Since no exact definition was available at that time regarding the metabolic syndrome, the authors [124] reasoned to examine the association of LDL size and pattern to specific insulin, proinsulin, increased triglyceride, decreased HDL, hypertension and impaired glucose tolerance in 488 non-diabetic subjects. They found that LDL size decreased in a stepwise fashion with increasing number of the metabolic disorders described above (zero 262.6 +/- 9.4; one 257.0 +/- 9.3; two 256.4 +/- 9.4; three 249.0 +/- 9.1; and four 244.9 +/- 9.0). These results were similar in men and women and in non-Hispanic whites and Mexican Americans. Notably, the association between LDL size and the number of metabolic disorders remained statistically significant even after adjustment for obesity, body fat distribution, gender, ethnicity, proinsulin and insulin concentrations.

Other studies [125,126] have more recently indirectly assessed the levels of small, dense LDL in subjects with the metabolic syndrome, using recent evidences that support the use of the triglyceride/HDL-cholesterol ratio for the prediction of LDL pattern B [127,128]. Many issues on the accuracy may be questioned, but this indirect measure holds the great advantages to be inexpensive as well as to be used in routine practice.

In summary, LDL size and subclasses show specific alterations in patients with the metabolic syndrome that probably significantly increase their cardiovascular risk; however, so far it has not been recommended by the international scientific societies to incorporate LDL size measurements in treatment plans, when hypolipidemic therapies are installed. However, measurements beyond traditional lipids, such as on the presence of small, dense LDL in patients with the metabolic syndrome, may help to identify cardiovascular risk subgroups. In addition, it might be possible in the future to individualize hypolipidemic treatments if more than the traditional lipids are taken into account. Particularly LDL size measurements may help to assess cardiovascular risk within the metabolic syndrome and adapt the treatment goals thereafter.

Therapeutic Modulation of LDL Subclasses: Effects of Statins and Fibrates

Hypolipidemic treatment is able of altering LDL subclass distribution and statins and fibrates are currently the most widely used lipid-lowering agents. Statins are potent inhibitors of hydroxy-methyl-glutaryl-coenzyme A reductase, the rate-limiting enzyme in hepatic cholesterol synthesis and are the primary drugs of choice for the treatment of elevated plasma LDL cholesterol concentrations. Fibrates have a major impact on triglyceride metabolism mediated by peroxisomal proliferation activator receptors (PPAR) and through stimulation of lipoprotein lipase [18].

Statins potentially lower large, medium and small LDL particles, but a strong variation has been noticed among the different agents. Treatment with pravastatin favorably altered the LDL size in four studies [129-132], but in others did not [133-144]. Similarly, simvastatin therapy showed significant [145-150], moderate [151,152] or no effect [153-164] on LDL subclasses. Yet, fluvastatin and atorvastatin seem to be more effective. Fluvastatin favorably altered the LDL size in six studies [165-170], but in two did not [171,172].

Treatment with atorvastatin resulted more frequently in a beneficial effect [144,149,173-188] than not [164,189-198]. Promising data were also recently published on the use of rosuvastatin [199]. Regarding fibrates, this class of hypolipidemic drug seems to be more powerful than statins on LDL size; in fact, therapy with fenofibrate, bezafibrate and gemfibrozil usually results in a beneficial effect [140,141,147,149,157,158,185,189,191,200-216], with very rare negative findings [153,217].

As already reported [18], although not directly demonstrated, the modulation of LDL size with fibrates probably contributed to the reduction of CHD risk in the "Helsinki Heart Study" and in the "Veterans Affairs High-density Lipoprotein Cholesterol Intervention Trials Study Group" [218-220]; in addition, it is likely that there was a bias towards small LDL in clinical trials that showed cardiovascular benefit from statins [221-223].

The Clinical Relevance of LDL Size Modulation

Other studies have more interestingly investigated if the therapeutic modification of LDL particle size by statins is significantly associated with reduced cardiovascular risk Such investigations used arteriographic changes as outcome variables and have reported that CAD progression in the control group is significantly greater in patients with a predominance of small, dense LDL [224] and that arteriographic benefit is concentrated in patients with a predominance of small, dense LDL who received treatment that tends to lower small dense LDL. These studies included the "Stanford Coronary Risk Intervention Project" (SCRIP), the "Familial Atherosclerosis Treatment Study" (FATS) and the "Pravastatin Limitation of Atherosclerosis in the Coronary Arteries" (PLAC-I) trial [225-227]. Lovastatin was admistered in the SCRIP (with bile acid-binding resins, niacin or fibrates) and in the FATS (with colestipol, versus niacin and colestipol), pravastin was used in the PLAC-I.

The therapeutical modulation of LDL size was significantly associated with reduced CHD risk in these three studies at univariate analysis. In addition, at multivariate analyses with adjustments for confounding factors, changes in LDL size by drug therapy were the best correlates of changes in coronary stenosis in FATS [226]. In PLAC-I, using a logistic regression models that adjusted for lipid levels and other confounding factors, elevated levels of small LDL were associated with a nine-fold increased risk of CAD progression, but only in the placebo group [227]. All these data seem to suggest that the therapeutic modification of LDL size is significantly associated with reduced cardiovascular risk, even after multivariate adjustment for confounding factors. However further studies are needed, in particular to test if specific lipid-lowering therapies are more beneficial in pattern B subjects versus those with pattern A [228-231].

Conclusions

Small, dense LDL are associated with increased risk for cardiovascular disease and diabetes mellitus and a reduction in LDL size has been reported in patients with acute myocardial infarction, with angina pectoris as well as in patients with non-coronary forms of atherosclerosis. LDL size seems also to be an important predictor of cardiovascular events and progression of coronary artery disease and the predominance of small dense LDL has been accepted as an emerging cardiovascular risk factor by the National Cholesterol Education Program Adult Treatment Panel III [3,10,16,19,232,233]. In addition, small, dense LDL, with elevated triglyceride levels and low HDL-cholesterol concentrations, constitute the "atherogenic lipoprotein phenotype" [9-11], a form of atherogenic dyslipidemia that is a feature of type 2 diabetes and the metabolic syndrome [3,8].

As recently stated by the joint American Heart Association/National Heart, Lung, and Blood Institute Scientific Statement on Diagnosis and Management of the Metabolic Syndrome, "atherogenic dyslipidemia can become a target for lipid-lowering therapy after the goal for LDL-cholesterol has been attained. In other words, as long as LDL-cholesterol remains above goal level, LDL-cholesterol is the primary target of therapy even in the metabolic syndrome" [8].

However, this point is still on debate, since this approach may leave substantial excess risk for cardiovascular disease in patients with this type of dyslipidemia [11,13,234]. As recently reported [234], even if modification of the atherogenic lipid triad is probably one of the most effective methods of reducing cardiovascular risk, therapy for atherogenic dyslipidemia is often directed to first lowering serum LDL-cholesterol levels, usually by statins. However, the results of recent trials evaluating statins have been mixed, even showing no significant effect on cardiovascular outcomes in subgroups of patients with diabetes and the recent Collaborative Atorvastatin Diabetes Study showed that atorvastatin can reduce cardiovascular events in a trial specifically designed for a diabetic population, though the population had to have at least one other risk factor in addition to diabetes [235].

By contrast, fibrates are potentially well suited to the treatment of dyslipidemia associated with type 2 diabetes and the metabolic syndrome, as they are usually more effective than statins for normalizing serum levels of HDL-cholesterol and triglycerides

[234]. In addition, fibrates are much more effective,compared to statins, in modifying LDL size and subclasses towards less atherogenic particles [18]. Promising results have been obtained from several trials using fibrates, such as the Bezafibrate Infarction Prevention study [236] and the Veterans Affairs Cooperative Studies Program HDL-C Intervention Trial (with gemfibrozil) [220]. In addition, new findings are available from the recent published Fenofibrate Intervention and Event Lowering in Diabetes (FIELD) trial [237], a clinical outcomes trial specifically designed to evaluate fenofibrate in a large population of patients with type 2 diabetes, many of whom have the metabolic syndrome. This multinational, randomised controlled trial included 9,795 participants aged 50-75 years, all with type 2 diabetes mellitus, and not taking statin therapy at study entry. The primary outcome was coronary events (coronary heart disease death or non-fatal myocardial infarction); the secondary outcome was total cardiovascular events (the composite of cardiovascular death, myocardial infarction, stroke, and coronary and carotid revascularization). The results of study were somehow disappointing: fenofibrate did not significantly reduce the risk of the primary outcome of coronary events and reduced only total cardiovascular events, mainly due to fewer non-fatal myocardial infarctions and revascularizations. However, it has to be emphasized that a very large portion of patients with the atherogenic lipoprotein phenotype was excluded according to the inclusion criteria of study: total-cholesterol concentration of 3.0-6.5 mmol/L and a total-cholesterol/HDL-cholesterol ratio of 4.0 or more or plasma triglyceride of 1.0-5.0 mmol/L. In other words, this study unfortunately excluded exactly the type of patients that would benefit most from fibrate therapy.

In conclusion, LDL size and subclasses show peculiar alterations in patients with the metabolic syndrome that probably significantly increase their cardiovascular risk; however, so far it is not recommended by the international scientific societies to treat such alterations with lipid-lowering molecules or with other agents. However, measurements beyond traditional lipids, such as on the presence of small, dense LDL in patients with the metabolic syndrome, may help to identify cardiovascular risk subgroups and it has been recently suggested that patients at very high cardiovascular risk should be managed carefully and potentially treated more aggressively [238].

To justify the routine measurement of LDL size, large clinical endpoint studies are necessary; these studies should investigate whether certain pharmacological therapies are more effective in reducing cardiovascular morbidity and mortality in pattern B compared to pattern A patients, independently from LDL-cholesterol. Therefore, it might be possible in the future to individualize hypolipidemic treatments if more than the traditional lipids are taken into account. Particularly LDL size measurements may help to assess cardiovascular risk within the metabolic syndrome and adapt the treatment goals thereafter.

Acknowledgements

The authors are grateful for the guidance and support provided over the years by Prof. Ronald M. Krauss (Senior Scientist, Lawrence Berkeley National Laboratory, University of California, Berkeley, USA and Director of Atherosclerosis Research, Children's Hospital Oakland Research Institute, Oakland, California, USA) and Prof. Alberto Notarbartolo

(Head, Department of Clinical Medicine and Emerging Diseases, University of Palermo, Italy). Kaspar Berneis was supported by a research grant from the Swiss National Foundation 3200B0-105258/1.

References

[1]   World Health Organization: Definition, Diagnosis, and Classification of Diabetes Mellitus and its Complications: Report of a WHO Consultation. *Geneva, World Health Org.*, 1999

[2]   Balkau B, Charles MA. Comment on the provisional report from the WHO consultation. European Group for the Study of Insulin Resistance (EGIR). *Diabet Med.* 1999;16:442– 443.

[3]   National Cholesterol Education Program (NCEP) Expert Panel on Detection, Evaluation, and Treatment of High Blood Cholesterol in Adults (Adult Treatment Panel III). Third Report of the National Cholesterol Education Program (NCEP) Expert Panel on Detection, Evaluation, and Treatment of High Blood Cholesterol in Adults (Adult Treatment Panel III) final report. *Circulation.* 2002;106:3143–3421.

[4]   Einhorn D, Reaven GM, Cobin RH, Ford E, Ganda OP, Handelsman Y, Hellman R, Jellinger PS, Kendall D, Krauss RM, Neufeld ND, Petak SM, Rodbard HW, Seibel JA, Smith DA, Wilson PW. American College of Endocrinology position statement on the insulin resistance syndrome. *Endocr. Pract.* 2003;9:237–252.

[5]   Grundy SM, Brewer HB Jr, Cleeman JI, Smith SC Jr., Lenfant C; American Heart Association; National Heart, Lung, and Blood Institute. Definition of metabolic syndrome: report of the National Heart, Lung, and Blood Institute/American Heart Association conference on scientific issues related to definition. *Circulation.* 2004;109:433– 438.

[6]   International Diabetes Federation. Worldwide definition of the metabolic syndrome. Available at: http://www.idf.org/webdata/docs/IDF_Metasyndrome_definition.pdf

[7]   Kahn R, Buse J, Ferrannini E, Stern M; American Diabetes Association; European Association for the Study of Diabetes. The metabolic syndrome: time for a critical appraisal: joint statement from the American Diabetes Association and the European Association for the Study of Diabetes. *Diabetes Care.* 2005; 28:2289-304.

[8]   Grundy SM, Cleeman JI, Daniels SR, Donato KA, Eckel RH, Franklin BA, Gordon DJ, Krauss RM, Savage PJ, Smith SC Jr, Spertus JA, Costa F; American Heart Association; National Heart, Lung, and Blood Institute. Diagnosis and management of the metabolic syndrome: an American Heart Association/National Heart, Lung, and Blood Institute Scientific Statement. *Circulation.* 2005; 112:2735-52.

[9]   Austin MA, King MC, Vranizan KM, Krauss RM. Atherogenic lipoprotein phenotype. A proposed genetic marker for coronary heart disease risk. Circulation 1990; 82: 495-506.

[10]   Krauss RM. Dietary and genetic probes of atherogenic dyslipidemia. *Arterioscler. Thromb. Vasc. Biol.* 2005; 25:2265-2272.

[11] Rizzo M and Berneis K. Lipid triad or atherogenic lipoprotein phenotype: a role in cardiovascular prevention ? *J. Atheroscl. Thromb.* 2005; 12:237-9.

[12] Sattar N, Petrie JR, Jaap AJ. The atherogenic lipoprotein phenotype and vascular endothelial dysfunction. *Atherosclerosis* 1998; 138: 229-35

[13] Superko HR. Beyond LDL cholesterol reduction. *Circulation* 1996; 94: 2351–4.

[14] Krauss RM and Blanche PJ. Detection and quantitation of LDL subfractions. *Curr. Opin. Lipidol.* 1992; 3:377-383.

[15] Packard C, Caslake M, Shepherd J. The role of small, dense low density lipoprotein (LDL): a new look. *Int. J. Card.* 2000; 74:S17–S22

[16] Berneis KK and Krauss RM. Metabolic origins and clinical significance of LDL heterogeneity. *J. Lipid. Res.* 2002; 43: 1363-1379.

[17] Berneis K and Rizzo M. LDL size: does it matter? *Swiss Med. Weekly.* 2004; 134:720–724.

[18] Rizzo M, Berneis K. Low-density-lipoproteins size and cardiovascular risk assessment *QJM – Int. J. Med.* 2006; 99: 1-14.

[19] Rizzo M and Berneis K. Should we measure routinely the LDL peak particle size? *Int. J. Card.* 2006; 107: 147-151.

[20] Krauss RM and Burke DJ. Identification of multiple subclasses of plasma low density lipoproteins in normal humans. *J. Lipid. Res.* 1982; 23:97-104.

[21] Krauss RM, Hellerstein MK, Neese RA, Blanche PJ, La Belle M, Shames DM: Altered metabolism of large low density lipoproteins in subjects with predominance of small low density lipoproteins. *Circulation* 92:1-102, 1995

[22] Rizzo M, Taylor JM, Barbagallo CM, Berneis K, Blanche PJ, Krauss RM: Effects on lipoprotein subclasses of combined expression of human hepatic lipase and human apoB in transgenic rabbits. *Arterioscler. Thromb. Vasc. Biol.* 24:141-146, 2004

[23] Sacks FM and Campos H. Low-Density Lipoprotein Size and Cardiovascular Disease: A Reappraisal. *J. Clin. Endocr. Metab.* 2003; 88:4525–4532.

[24] Rizzo M, Barbagallo CM, Severino M, Polizzi F, Onorato F, Noto D, Cefalù AB, Pace A, G Marino, Notarbartolo A, Averna RM. Low-density-lipoproteins particle size in a population living in a small mediterranean island. *Eur. J. Clin. Invest.* 2003; 33:126-133.

[25] Bjornheden T, Babyi A, Bondjers G, Wiklund O. Accumulation of lipoprotein fractions and subfractions in the arterial wall, determined in an in vitro perfusion system. *Atherosclerosis* 1996; 123:43-56.

[26] Galeano NF, Al-Haideri M, Keyserman F, Rumsey SC, Deckelbaum RJ. Small dense low density lipoprotein has increased affinity for LDL receptor-independent cell surface binding sites: a potential mechanism for increased atherogenicity. *J. Lipid. Res.* 1998; 39:1263-1273.

[27] Camejo G, Lopez A, Lopez F, Quinones J. Interaction of low density lipoproteins with arterial proteoglycans. The role of charge and sialic acid content. *Atherosclerosis* 1985; 55:93-105.

[28] Tribble DL, Rizzo M, Chait A, Lewis DM, Blanche PJ, Krauss RM. Enhanced oxidative susceptibility and reduced antioxidant content of metabolic precursors of small, dense low-density lipoproteins. *Am. J. Med.* 2001; 110:103-110.

[29] Tribble DL, Holl LG, Wood PD, Krauss RM. Variations in oxidative susceptibility among six low density lipoprotein subfractions of differing density and particle size. *Atherosclerosis* 1992; 93:189-199.

[30] de Graaf J, Hak-Lemmers HL, Hectors MP, Demacker PN, Hendriks JC, Stalenhoef AF. Enhanced susceptibility to in vitro oxidation of the dense low density lipoprotein subfraction in healthy subjects. *Arterioscler. Thromb.* 1991; 11:298-306.

[31] Berneis K, Shames DM, Blanche PJ, La Belle M, Rizzo M, Krauss RM. Plasma clearance of human low-density lipoprotein in human apolipoprotein B transgenic mice is related to particle diameter. *Metabolism* 2004; 53:483-487.

[32] Crouse JR, Parks JS, Schey HM, Kahl FR. Studies of low density lipoprotein molecular weight in human beings with coronary artery disease. *J. Lipid. Res.* 1985; 26:566–574

[33] Austin MA, Breslow JL, Hennekens CH, Buring JE, Willett WC, Krauss RM. Low-density lipoprotein subclass patterns and risk of myocardial infarction. *JAMA* 1988; 260:1917–1921

[34] Griffin BA, Caslake MJ, Yip B, Tait GW, Packard CJ, Shepherd J. Rapid isolation of low density lipoprotein (LDL) subfractions from plasma by density gradient ultracentrifugation. *Atherosclerosis* 1990; 83:59-67.

[35] Tornvall P, Karpe F, Carlson LA, Hamsten A. Relationships of low density lipoprotein subfractions to angiographically defined coronary disease in young survivors of myocardial infarction. *Atherosclerosis* 1991; 90:67–80

[36] Campos H, Genest J, Blijlevens E, McNamara JR, Jenner JL, Ordovas JM, Wilson PW, Schaefer EJ. Low density lipoprotein particle size and coronary artery disease. *Arteriosclerosis* 1992; 12:187–195

[37] Coresh J, Kwiterovich Jr PO, Smith HH, Bachorik PS. Association of plasma triglyceride concentration and LDL particle diameter, density, and chemical composition with premature coronary artery disease in men and women. *J. Lipid. Res.* 1993; 34:1687–1697

[38] Griffin BA, Freeman DJ, Tait GW, Thomson J, Caslake MJ, Packard CJ, Shepherd J. Role of plasma triglyceride in the regulation of plasma low density lipoprotein (LDL) subfractions: relative contribution of small dense LDL to coronary heart disease risk. *Atherosclerosis* 1994; 106:241–253.

[39] Campos H, Roederer GO, Lussier-Cacan S, Davignon J, Krauss RM. Predominance of large LDL and reduced HDL2 cholesterol in normolipidemic with coronary artery disease. *Arterioscler. Thromb. Vasc. Biol.* 1995; 15:1043–1048

[40] Sherrard B, Simpson H, Cameron J, Wahi S, Jennings G, Dart A. LDL particle size in subjects with previously unsuspected coronary heart disease: relationship with other cardiovascular risk markers. *Atherosclerosis* 1996; 126:277–287

[41] Rajman I, Kendall MJ, Cramb R, Holder RL, Salih M, Gammage MD. Investigation of low density lipoprotein subfractions as a coronary risk factor in normotriglyceridaemic men. *Atherosclerosis* 1996; 125:231–242

[42] Stampfer MJ, Krauss RM, Ma J, Blanche PJ, Holl LG, Sacks FM, Hennekens CH. A study of triglyceride level, low-density lipoprotein particle diameter, and risk of myocardial infarction. *JAMA* 1996; 276:882–88.

[43] Gardner CD, Fortmann SP, Krauss RM. Association of small low-density lipoprotein particles with the incidence of coronary artery disease in men and women. *JAMA* 1996; 276:875–881

[44] Miller BD, Alderman EL, Haskell WL, Fair JM, Krauss RM. Predominance of dense low-density lipoprotein particles predicts angiographic benefit of therapy in the Stanford Coronary Risk Intervention Project. *Circulation* 1996; 94:2146–2153

[45] Mack WJ, Krauss RM, Hodis HN Lipoprotein subclasses in the Monitored Atherosclerosis Regression Study (MARS). Treatment effects and relation to coronary angiographic progression. *Arterioscler. Thromb. Vasc. Biol.* 1996; 16:697–704

[46] Lamarche B, Tchernof A, Moorjani S, Cantin B, Dagenais GR, Lupien PJ, Despres JP. Small, dense low-density lipoprotein particles as a predictor of the risk of ischemic heart disease in men. P results from the Quebec Cardiovascular Study. *Circulation* 1997; 95:69–75

[47] Gray RS, Robbins DC, Wang W, Yeh JL, Fabsitz RR, Cowan LD, Welty TK, Lee ET, Krauss RM, Howard BV. Relation of LDL size to the insulin resistance syndrome and coronary heart disease in American Indians. The Strong Heart Study. *Arterioscler Thromb. Vasc. Biol.* 1997; 17:2713–2720

[48] Wahi S, Gatzka CD, Sherrard B, Simpson H, Collins V, Dowse G, Zimmet P, Jennings G, Dart AM. Risk factors for coronary heart disease in a population with a high prevalence of obesity and diabetes: a case-control study of the Polynesian population of Western Samoa. *J. Cardiovasc. Risk.* 1997; 4:173–178.

[49] Slyper AH, Zvereva S, Schectman G, Hoffmann RG, Walker JA. Lowdensity lipoprotein particle size is not a discriminating marker for atherogenic risk in male offspring of parents with early coronary artery disease. *Metabolism* 1997; 46:954–958

[50] Freedman DS, Otvos JD, Jeyarajah EJ, Barboriak JJ, Anderson AJ, Walker JA. Relation of lipoprotein subclasses as measured by proton nuclear magnetic resonance spectroscopy to coronary artery disease. *Arterioscler. Thromb. Vasc. Biol.* 1998; 18:1046-53.

[51] Ruotolo G, Ericsson CG, Tettamanti C, Karpe F, Grip L, Svane B, Nilsson J, de Faire U, Hamsten A. Treatment effects on serum lipoprotein lipids, apolipoproteins and low density lipoprotein particle size and relationships of lipoprotein variables to progression of coronary artery disease in the Bezafibrate Coronary Atherosclerosis Intervention Trial (BECAIT). *J. Am. Coll. Cardiol.* 1998; 32:1648-56.

[52] O'Neal DN, Lewicki J, Ansari MZ, et al. Lipid levels and peripheral vascular disease in diabetic and non-diabetic subjects. *Atherosclerosis* 1998;136:1-8.

[53] Landray MJ, Sagar G, Muskin J, Murray S, Holder RL, Lip GYH. Association of atherogenic low-density lipoprotein subfractions with carotid atherosclerosis. *Q. J. Med.* 1998; 91:345–351

[54] Hulthe J, Wiklund O, Olsson G, Fagerberg B, Bokemark L, Nivall S, Wikstrand J. Computerized measurement of LDL particle size in human serum. Reproducibility studies and evaluation of LDL particle size in relation to metabolic variables and the occurrence of atherosclerosis. *Scand. J. Clin. Lab. Invest.* 1999;59:649-61.

[55] Mykkanen L, Kuusisto J, Haffner S, Laakso M, AustinMA. LDL size and risk of coronary heart disease in elderly men and women. *Arterioscler. Thromb. Vasc. Biol.* 1999; 19:2742-2748

[56] Erbey JR, Robbins D, Forrest KY, Orchard TJ. Low-density lipoprotein particle size and coronary artery disease in a childhood-onset type 1 diabetes population. *Metabolism.* 1999; 48:531-4.

[57] Skoglund-Andersson C, Tang R, Bond MG, de Faire U, Hamsten A, Karpe F LDL particle size distribution is associated with carotid intima-media thickness in healthy 50-year-old men. *Arterioscler. Thromb. Vasc. Biol.* 1999; 19:2422-2430

[58] Zambon A, Hokanson JE, Brown BG, Brunzell JD. Evidence for a new pathophysiological mechanism for coronary artery disease regression: hepatic lipase-mediated changes in LDL density. *Circulation* 1999; 99:1959-64.

[59] Austin MA, Rodriguez BL, McKnight B, McNeely MJ, Edwards KL, Curb JD, Sharp DS 2000 Low-density lipoprotein particle size, triglycerides, and highdensity lipoprotein cholesterol as risk factors for coronary heart disease in older Japanese-American men. *Am. J. Cardiol.* 86:412–416

[60] Hulthe J, Wiklund O, Bondjers G, Wikstrand J 2000 LDL particle size in relation to intima-media thickness and plaque occurrence in the carotid and femoral arteries in patients with hypercholesterolaemia. *J. Intern. Med.* 248:42–52

[61] Hulthe J, Bokemark L, Wikstrand J, Fagerberg B. The metabolic syndrome, LDL particle size, and atherosclerosis: the Atherosclerosis and Insulin Resistance (AIR) study. *Arterioscler. Thromb. Vasc. Biol.* 2000; 20:2140–2147.

[62] Bokemark L, Wikstrand J, Attvall S, Hulthe J, Wedel H, Fagerberg B. Insulin resistance and intima-media thickness in the carotid and femoral arteries of clinically healthy 58-year-old men. The Atherosclerosis and Insulin Resistance Study (AIR). *J. Intern. Med.* 2001; 249:59-67.

[63] Campos H, Moye LA, Glasser SP, Stampfer MJ, Sacks FM. Low-density lipoprotein size, pravastatin treatment, and coronary events. *JAMA* 2001; 286:1468–1474

[64] Kamigaki AS, Siscovick DS, Schwartz SM, Psaty BM, Edwards KL, Raghunathan TE, Austin MA. Low density lipoprotein particle size and risk of early-onset myocardial infarction in women. *Am. J. Epidemiol.* 2001; 153:939–945

[65] Rosenson RS, Otvos JD, Freedman DS. Relations of lipoprotein subclass levels and low-density lipoprotein size to progression of coronary artery disease in the Pravastatin Limitation of Atherosclerosis in the Coronary Arteries (PLAC-I) trial. *Am. J. Cardiol.* 2002; 90:89–94

[66] Blake GJ, Otvos JD, Rifai N, Ridker PM. Low-density lipoprotein particle concentration and size as determined by nuclear magnetic resonance spectroscopy as predictors of cardiovascular disease in women. *Circulation* 2002; 106:1930–1937

[67] Kuller L, Arnold A, Tracy R, Otvos J, Burke G, Psaty B, Siscovick D, Freedman DS, Kronmal R. Nuclear magnetic resonance spectroscopy of lipoproteins and risk of coronary heart disease in the cardiovascular health study. *Arterioscler. Thromb. Vasc. Biol.* 2002; 22:1175–1180

[68] Liu ML, Ylitalo K, Nuotio I, Salonen R, Salonen JT, Taskinen MR. Association between carotid intima-media thickness and low-density lipoprotein size and

susceptibility of low-density lipoprotein to oxidation in asymptomatic members of familial combined hyperlipidemia families. *Stroke* 2002; 33:1255–1260

[69] Koba S, Hirano T, Kondo T, Shibata M, Suzuki H, Murakami M, Geshi E, Katagiri T. Significance of small dense low-density lipoproteins and other risk factors in patients with various types of coronary heart disease. *Am. Heart. J.* 2002; 144:1026-35.

[70] Vakkilainen J, Pajukanta P, Cantor RM, Nuotio IO, Lahdenpera S, Ylitalo K, Pihlajamaki J, Kovanen PT, Laakso M, Viikari JS, Peltonen L, Taskinen MR. Genetic influences contributing to LDL particle size in familial combined hyperlipidaemia. *Eur. J. Hum. Genet.* 2002; 10:547-52.

[71] Slowik A, Iskra T, Turaj W, Hartwich J, Dembinska-Kiec A, Szczudlik A. LDL phenotype B and other lipid abnormalities in patients with large vessel disease and small vessel disease. *Neurol. Sci.* 2003; 214:11-6.

[72] Hallman DM, Brown SA, Ballantyne CM, Sharrett AR, Boerwinkle E. Relationship between low-density lipoprotein subclasses and asymptomatic atherosclerosis in subjects from the Atherosclerosis Risk in Communities (ARIC) Study. *Biomarkers.* 2004; 9:190-202.

[73] Watanabe T, Koba S, Kawamura M, Itokawa M, Idei T, Nakagawa Y, Iguchi T, Katagiri T. Small dense low-density lipoprotein and carotid atherosclerosis in relation to vascular dementia. *Metabolism.* 2004; 53:476-82.

[74] Wallenfeldt K, Bokemark L, Wikstrand J, Hulthe J, Fagerberg B. Apolipoprotein B/apolipoprotein A-I in relation to the metabolic syndrome and change in carotid artery intima-media thickness during 3 years in middle-aged men. *Stroke.* 2004;35:2248-52.

[75] Kullo IJ, Bailey KR, McConnell JP, Peyser PA, Bielak LF, Kardia SL, Sheedy PF 2nd, Boerwinkle E, Turner ST. Low-density lipoprotein particle size and coronary atherosclerosis in subjects belonging to hypertensive sibships. *Am. J. Hypertens.* 2004; 17:845-51.

[76] van Tits LJ, Smilde TJ, van Wissen S, de Graaf J, Kastelein JJ, Stalenhoef AF. Effects of atorvastatin and simvastatin on low-density lipoprotein subfraction profile, low-density lipoprotein oxidizability, and antibodies to oxidized low-density lipoprotein in relation to carotid intima media thickness in familial hypercholesterolemia. *J Investig Med.* 2004;52:177-84.

[77] Inukai T, Yamamoto R, Suetsugu M, Matsumoto S, Wakabayashi S, Inukai Y, Matsutomo R, Takebayashi K, Aso Y. Small low-density lipoprotein and small low-density lipoprotein/total low-density lipoprotein are closely associated with intima-media thickness of the carotid artery in Type 2 diabetic patients. *J. Diabetes. Complications.* 2005; 19:269-75.

[78] Mohan V, Deepa R, Velmurugan K, Gokulakrishnan K. Association of small dense LDL with coronary artery disease and diabetes in urban Asian Indians - the Chennai Urban Rural Epidemiology Study (CURES-8). *J. Assoc. Physicians India.* 2005; 53:95-100.

[79] Yoon Y, Song J, Park HD, Park KU, Kim JQ. Significance of small dense low-density lipoproteins as coronary risk factor in diabetic and non-diabetic Korean populations. *Clin. Chem. Lab. Med.* 2005; 43:431-7.

[80] St-Pierre AC, Cantin B, Dagenais GR, Mauriege P, Bernard PM, Despres JP, Lamarche B. Low-density lipoprotein subfractions and the long-term risk of ischemic heart disease in men: 13-year follow-up data from the Quebec Cardiovascular Study. *Arterioscler. Thromb. Vasc. Biol.* 2005;25:553-9.

[81] Berneis K, Jeanneret C, Muser J, Felix B, Miserez AR. Low-density lipoprotein size and subclasses are markers of clinically apparent and non-apparent atherosclerosis in type 2 diabetes. *Metabolism.* 2005;54:227-234.

[82] Otvos JD, Freedman DS, Pegus C. *LDL and HDL particle subclasses are independent predictors of cardiovascular events in Veteran Affairs HDL Intervention Trial (VA-HIT).* Paper presented at the AHA Annual Scientific Session. Chicago, USA, 2002.

[83] Lada AT, Rudel LL. Associations of low density lipoprotein particle composition with atherogenicity. *Curr. Opin. Lipidol.* 2004; 15:19-24.

[84] Lamarche B, Lemieux I, Despres JP. The small, dense LDL phenotype and the risk of coronary heart disease: epidemiology, patho-physiology and therapeutic aspects. *Diabetes Metab.* 1999; 25:199-211.

[85] Rader DJ, Hoeg JM, Brewer HB Jr. Quantitation of plasma apolipoproteins in the primary and secondary prevention of coronary artery disease. *Ann. Intern. Med.* 1994;120: 1012-25.

[86] Sniderman AD, Furberg CD, Keech A, Roeters van Lennep JE, Frohlich J, Jungner I, Walldius G. Apolipoproteins versus lipids as indices of coronary risk and as targets for statin treatment. *Lancet* 2003; 361:777-80.

[87] Cromwell WC, Otvos JD. Low-density lipoprotein particle number and risk for cardiovascular disease. *Curr. Atheroscler. Rep.* 2004; 6:381-7.

[88] Garvey WT, Kwon S, Zheng D, Shaughnessy S, Wallace P, Hutto A, Pugh K, Jenkins AJ, Klein RL, Liao Y. Effects of insulin resistance and type 2 diabetes on lipoprotein subclass particle size and concentration determined by nuclear magnetic resonance. *Diabetes* 2003; 52:453-62.

[89] Otvos J, Cronwell W, Shalaurova I. LDL particle but not LDL cholesterol are highly elevated in the metabolic syndrome. Results from the Framingham Offspring Study. *Circulation* 2003; 108:IV-740. (abstract)

[90] Avogaro P, Bon GB, Cazzolato G et al. Variations in apolipoproteins B and A1 during the course of myocardial infarction. *Eur. J. Clin. Invest.* 1978 ; 8 : 121-9.

[91] Rosenson RS. Myocardial injury: the acute phase response and lipoprotein metabolism. *J. Am. Coll. Cardiol.* 1993; 22: 933-40.

[92] Carlsson R, Lindberg G, Westin L, Israelsson B: Serum lipids four weeks after acute myocardial infarction are a valid basis for lipid lowering intervention in patients receiving thrombolysis. *Br. Heart. J.* 1995; 74: 18-20.

[93] Kingswood JC, Williams S, Owens DR. How soon after myocardial infarction should plasma lipid values be assessed? *Br. Med. J.* 1984; 289: 1651-3.

[94] Barbagallo CM, Rizzo M, Cefalù AB et al. Changes in plasma lipids and low-density lipoprotein peak particle size during and after myocardial infarction. *Am. J. Card.* 2002; 89: 460-2.

[95] Miwa K. Low density lipoprotein particles are small in patients with coronary vasospasm. *Int. J. Cardiol.* 2003; 87:193-201.

[96] Leonsson M, Hulthe J, Oscarsson J, Johannsson G, Wendelhag I, Wikstrand J, Bengtsson BA. Intima-media thickness in cardiovascularly asymptomatic hypopituitary adults with growth hormone deficiency: relation to body mass index, gender, and other cardiovascular risk factors. *Clin. Endocrinol. (Oxf).* 2002;57:751-9.

[97] Raal FJ, Pilcher GJ, Waisberg R, Buthelezi EP, Veller MG, Joffe BI. Low-density lipoprotein cholesterol bulk is the pivotal determinant of atherosclerosis in familial hypercholesterolemia. *Am. J. Cardiol.* 1999;83:1330-3.

[98] Lupattelli G, Pasqualini L, Siepi D, Marchesi S, Pirro M, Vaudo G, Ciuffetti G, Mannarino E. Increased postprandial lipemia in patients with normolipemic peripheral arterial disease. *Am. Heart. J.* 2002; 143:733-8.

[99] Gorter PM, Olijhoek JK, van der Graaf Y, Algra A, Rabelink TJ, Visseren FL; SMART Study Group. Prevalence of the metabolic syndrome in patients with coronary heart disease, cerebrovascular disease, peripheral arterial disease or abdominal aortic aneurysm. *Atherosclerosis.* 2004; 173:363-9.

[100] Reaven GM. Banting lecture. Role of insulin resistance in human disease. *Diabetes 37*:1595-607, 1988

[101] Selby JV, Austin MA, Newman B et al. LDL subclass phenotypes and the insulin resistance syndrome in women. *Circulation* 88:381-7, 1993

[102] Syvanne M, Taskinen MR. Lipids and lipoproteins as coronary risk factors in non-insulin- dependent diabetes mellitus. *Lancet 350 Suppl 1*:SI20-3, 1997

[103] U.K. Prospective Diabetes Study 27. Plasma Lipids and lipoproteins at diagnosis of NIDDM by age and sex. *Diabetes Care 20*:1683-7, 1997

[104] Friedlander Y, Kidron M, Caslake M, Lamb T, McConnell M, Bar-On H. Low density lipoprotein particle size and risk factors of insulin resistance syndrome. *Atherosclerosis 148*:141-9, 2000

[105] Austin MA, Mykkanen L, Kuusisto J et al. Prospective study of small LDLs as a risk factor for non-insulin dependent diabetes mellitus in elderly men and women. *Circulation 92*:1770-8, 1995

[106] Reaven GM, Chen YD, Jeppesen J, Maheux P, Krauss RM. Insulin resistance and hyperinsulinemia in individuals with small, dense low density lipoprotein particles. *J. Clin. Invest.* 1993;92:141–146.

[107] Feingold KR, Grunfeld C, Pang M, Doerrler W, Krauss RM. LDL subclass phenotypes and triglyceride metabolism in non-insulin-dependent diabetes. *Arterioscler. Thromb.* 1992; 12:1496-502.

[108] Chambless LE, Heiss G, Folsom AR et al. Association of coronary heart disease incidence with carotid arterial wall thickness and major risk factors: the Atherosclerosis Risk in Communities (ARIC) Study, 1987-1993. *Am. J. Epidemiol.* 146:483-94, 1997

[109] Craven TE, Ryu JE, Espeland MA et al. Evaluation of the associations between carotid artery atherosclerosis and coronary artery stenosis. A case-control study. *Circulation 82*:1230-42, 1990

[110] Salonen JT, Salonen R. Ultrasound B-mode imaging in observational studies of atherosclerotic progression. *Circulation 87*:II56-65, 1993

[111] Wofford JL, Kahl FR, Howard GR, McKinney WM, Toole JF, Crouse JR, 3rd. Relation of extent of extracranial carotid artery atherosclerosis as measured by B-mode

ultrasound to the extent of coronary atherosclerosis. *Arterioscler. Thromb. 11*:1786-94, 1991

[112] Goya K, Kitamura T, Inaba M, et al. Risk factors for asymptomatic atherosclerosis in Japanese type 2 diabetic patients without diabetic microvascular complications. *Metabolism 52*:1302-6, 2003

[113] Niskanen L, Rauramaa R, Miettinen H, Haffner SM, Mercuri M, Uusitupa M. Carotid artery intima-media thickness in elderly patients with NIDDM and in nondiabetic subjects. *Stroke 27*:1986-92, 1996

[114] Rizzo M, Barbagallo CM, Noto D, Pace A, Cefalu' AB, Pernice V, Rubino A, Pinto V, Pieri D, Traina M, Frasheri A, Notarbartolo A, Averna MR. Diabetes, family hystory and extension of coronary atherosclerosis are strong predictors of adverse events after PTCA: a one year follow-up study. *Nutrition, Metabolism and Cardiovascular Diseases*. 2005; 15:361-7.ù

[115] Carmina E, Lobo RA. Polycystic ovary syndrome (PCOS): arguably the most common endocrinopathy is associated with significant morbidity in women. *J Clin Endocrinol Metab*. 1999; 84:1897-9.

[116] Lobo RA, Carmina E. The importance of diagnosing the polycystic ovary syndrome. *Ann. Intern. Med.* 2000; 132:989-93.

[117] Rotterdam ESHRE/ASRM Sponsored PCOS Consensus Workshop Group. Revised 2003 consensus on diagnostic criteria and long-term health risks related to polycystic ovary syndrome. *Fertil. Steril.* 2004; 81:19-25.

[118] Carmina E, Rosato F, Jannì A, Rizzo M, Longo RA. Relative prevalence of different androgen excess disorders in 950 women referred because of clinical hyperandrogenism. *Journal of Cinical Endocinology and Metabolism* 2006; 91: 2-6.

[119] Guzick DS. Cardiovascular risk in PCOS. *J. Clin. Endocrinol. Metab.* 2004; 89:3694-5.

[120] Dejager S, Pichard C, Giral P, Bruckert E, Federspield MC, Beucler I, Turpin G. Smaller LDL particle size in women with polycystic ovary syndrome compared to controls. *Clin. Endocrinol. (Oxf)*. 2001 Apr;54(4):455-62.

[121] Pirwany IR, Fleming R, Greer IA, Packard CJ, Sattar N. Lipids and lipoprotein subfractions in women with PCOS: relationship to metabolic and endocrine parameters. *Clin. Endocrinol. (Oxf)*. 2001 Apr;54(4):447-53.

[122] Legro RS, Blanche P, Krauss RM, Lobo RA. Alterations in low-density lipoprotein and high-density lipoprotein subclasses among Hispanic women with polycystic ovary syndrome: influence of insulin and genetic factors. *Fertil. Steril.* 1999 Dec;72(6):990-5.

[123] Strowitzki T, Halser B, Demant T. Body fat distribution, insulin sensitivity, ovarian dysfunction and serum lipoproteins in patients with polycystic ovary syndrome. *Gynecol. Endocrinol.* 2002 Feb;16(1):45-51.

[124] Haffner SM, Mykkanen L, Robbins D, Valdez R, Miettinen H, Howard BV, Stern MP, Bowsher R. A preponderance of small dense LDL is associated with specific insulin, proinsulin and the components of the insulin resistance syndrome in non-diabetic subjects. *Diabetologia*. 1995; 38:1328-36.

[125] Garin MC, Kalix B, Morabia A, James RW. Small, dense lipoprotein particles and reduced paraoxonase-1 in patients with the metabolic syndrome. *J. Clin. Endocrinol. Metab.* 2005; 90:2264-9.

[126] Slapikas R, Luksiene D, Slapikiene B, Babarskiene MR, Grybauskiene R, Linoniene L. Prevalence of cardiovascular risk factors in coronary heart disease patients with different low-density lipoprotein phenotypes. *Medicina (Kaunas)*. 2005; 41:925-31.

[127] Hanak V, Munoz J, Teague J, Stanley A Jr, Bittner V. Accuracy of the triglyceride to high-density lipoprotein cholesterol ratio for prediction of the low-density lipoprotein phenotype B. *Am. J. Cardiol.* 2004; 94:219-22.

[128] McLaughlin T, Reaven G, Abbasi F, Lamendola C, Saad M, Waters D, Simon J, Krauss RM. Is there a simple way to identify insulin-resistant individuals at increased risk of cardiovascular disease? *Am. J. Cardiol.* 2005; 96:399-404.

[129] O'Keefe JH Jr, Harris WS, Nelson J, Windsor SL. Effects of pravastatin with niacin or magnesium on lipid levels and postprandial lipemia. *Am. J. Cardiol.* 1995;76(7):480-4.

[130] Otvos JD, Shalaurova I, Freedman DS, Rosenson RS. Effects of pravastatin treatment on lipoprotein subclass profiles and particle size in the PLAC-I trial. *Atherosclerosis*. 2002;160(1):41-8.

[131] Rosenson RS, Otvos JD, Freedman DS. Relations of lipoprotein subclass levels and low-density lipoprotein size to progression of coronary artery disease in the Pravastatin Limitation of Atherosclerosis in the Coronary Arteries (PLAC-I) trial. *Am. J. Cardiol.* 2002;90(2):89-94.

[132] Masana L, Villoria J, Sust M, Ros E, Plana N, Perez-Jimenez F, Franco M, Olivan JJ, Pinto X, Videla S. Treatment of type IIb familial combined hyperlipidemia with the combination pravastatin-piperazine sultosilate. *Eur. J. Pharmacol.* 2004 Aug 2;496(1-3):205-12.

[133] Vega GL, Krauss RM, Grundy SM. Pravastatin therapy in primary moderate hypercholesterolaemia: changes in metabolism of apolipoprotein B-containing lipoproteins. *J. Intern. Med.* 1990;227(2):81-94.

[134] Cheung MC, Austin MA, Moulin P, Wolf AC, Cryer D, Knopp RH. Effects of pravastatin on apolipoprotein-specific high density lipoprotein subpopulations and low density lipoprotein subclass phenotypes in patients with primary hypercholesterolemia. *Atherosclerosis*. 1993;102(1):107-19.

[135] Contacos C, Barter PJ, Sullivan DR. Effect of pravastatin and omega-3 fatty acids on plasma lipids and lipoproteins in patients with combined hyperlipidemia. *Arterioscler. Thromb.* 1993;13(12):1755-62.

[136] Zambon S, Cortella A, Sartore G, Baldo-Enzi G, Manzato E, Crepaldi G. Pravastatin treatment in combined hyperlipidaemia. Effect on plasma lipoprotein levels and size. *Eur. J. Clin. Pharmacol.*; 46(3):221-4.

[137] Franceschini G, Cassinotti M, Vecchio G, Gianfranceschi G, Pazzucconi F, Murakami T, Sirtori M, D'Acquarica AL, Sirtori CR. Pravastatin effectively lowers LDL cholesterol in familial combined hyperlipidemia without changing LDL subclass pattern. *Arterioscler. Thromb.* 1994;14(10):1569-75.

[138] Guerin M, Dolphin PJ, Talussot C, Gardette J, Berthezene F, Chapman MJ. Pravastatin modulates cholesteryl ester transfer from HDL to apoB-containing lipoproteins and lipoprotein subspecies profile in familial hypercholesterolemia. *Arterioscler. Thromb. Vasc. Biol.* 1995;15(9):1359-68.

[139] Contacos C, Barter PJ, Vrga L, Sullivan DR. Cholesteryl ester transfer in hypercholesterolaemia: fasting and postprandial studies with and without pravastatin. *Atherosclerosis.* 1998;141(1):87-98

[140] Rustemeijer C, Schouten JA, Voerman HJ, Hensgens HE, Donker AJ, Heine RJ. Pravastatin compared to bezafibrate in the treatment of dyslipidemia in insulin-treated patients with type 2 diabetes mellitus. *Diabetes. Metab. Res. Rev.* 2000;16(2):82-7.

[141] Lemieux I, Laperriere L, Dzavik V, Tremblay G, Bourgeois J, Despres JP. A 16-week fenofibrate treatment increases LDL particle size in type IIA dyslipidemic patients. *Atherosclerosis.* 2002;162(2):363-71.

[142] Blake GJ, Albert MA, Rifai N, Ridker PM. Effect of pravastatin on LDL particle concentration as determined by NMR spectroscopy: a substudy of a randomized placebo controlled trial. *Eur. Heart. J.* 2003;24(20):1843-7.

[143] Kazama H, Usui S, Okazaki M, Hosoi T, Ito H, Orimo H. Effects of bezafibrate and pravastatin on remnant-like lipoprotein particles and lipoprotein subclasses in type 2 diabetes. *Diabetes Res. Clin. Pract.* 2003;59(3):181-9.

[144] Sirtori CR, Calabresi L, Pisciotta L, Cattin L, Pauciullo P, Montagnani M, Manzato E, Bittolo Bon G, Fellin R. Effect of statins on LDL particle size in patients with familial combined hyperlipidemia: a comparison between atorvastatin and pravastatin. *Nutr. Metab. Cardiovasc. Dis.* 2005;15(1):47-55.

[145] Homma Y, Ozawa H, Kobayashi T, Yamaguchi H, Sakane H, Nakamura H. Effects of simvastatin on plasma lipoprotein subfractions, cholesterol esterification rate, and cholesteryl ester transfer protein in type II hyperlipoproteinemia. *Atherosclerosis.* 1995 Apr 24;114(2):223-34.

[146] Kontopoulos AG, Athyros VG, Papageorgiou AA, Hatzikonstandinou HA, Mayroudi MC, Boudoulas H. Effects of simvastatin and ciprofibrate alone and in combination on lipid profile, plasma fibrinogen and low density lipoprotein particle structure and distribution in patients with familial combined hyperlipidaemia and coronary artery disease. *Coron. Artery. Dis.* 1996 Nov;7(11):843-50.

[147] Nestel P, Simons L, Barter P, Clifton P, Colquhoun D, Hamilton-Craig I, Sikaris K, Sullivan D. A comparative study of the efficacy of simvastatin and gemfibrozil in combined hyperlipoproteinemia: prediction of response by baseline lipids, apo E genotype, lipoprotein(a) and insulin. *Atherosclerosis.* 1997 Mar 21;129(2):231-9.

[148] Forster LF, Stewart G, Bedford D, Stewart JP, Rogers E, Shepherd J, Packard CJ, Caslake MJ. Influence of atorvastatin and simvastatin on apolipoprotein B metabolism in moderate combined hyperlipidemic subjects with low VLDL and LDL fractional clearance rates. *Atherosclerosis.* 2002 Sep;164(1):129-45.

[149] Vega GL, Ma PT, Cater NB, Filipchuk N, Meguro S, Garcia-Garcia AB, Grundy SM. Effects of adding fenofibrate (200 mg/day) to simvastatin (10 mg/day) in patients with combined hyperlipidemia and metabolic syndrome. *J. Cardiol.* 2003 Apr 15;91(8):956-60.

[150] Bays HE, McGovern ME. Once-daily niacin extended release/lovastatin combination tablet has more favorable effects on lipoprotein particle size and subclass distribution than atorvastatin and simvastatin. *Prev. Cardiol.* 2003 Fall;6(4):179-88.

[151] Wakatsuki A, Ikenoue N, Izumiya C, Okatani Y, Sagara Y. Effect of estrogen and simvastatin on low-density lipoprotein subclasses in hypercholesterolemic postmenopausal women. *Obstet Gynecol.* 1998 Sep;92(3):367-72.

[152] Wakatsuki A, Okatani Y, Ikenoue N. Effects of combination therapy with estrogen plus simvastatin on lipoprotein metabolism in postmenopausal women with type IIa hypercholesterolemia. *Atherosclerosis.* 2000 May;150(1):103-11.

[153] Nakandakare E, Garcia RC, Rocha JC, Sperotto G, Oliveira HC, Quintao EC. Effects of simvastatin, bezafibrate and gemfibrozil on the quantity and composition of plasma lipoproteins. *Atherosclerosis.* 1990 Dec;85(2-3):211-7.

[154] Zhao SP, Hollaar L, van 't Hooft FM, Smelt AH, Gevers Leuven JA, van der Laarse A. Effect of simvastatin on the apparent size of LDL particles in patients with type IIB hyperlipoproteinemia. *Clin. Chim. Acta.* 1991 Dec 16;203(2-3):109-17.

[155] Gaw A, Packard CJ, Murray EF, Lindsay GM, Griffin BA, Caslake MJ, Vallance BD, Lorimer AR, Shepherd J. Effects of simvastatin on apoB metabolism and LDL subfraction distribution. *Arterioscler Thromb.* 1993 Feb;13(2):170-89.

[156] de Graaf J, Demacker PN, Stalenhoef AF. The effect of simvastatin treatment on the low-density lipoprotein subfraction profile and composition in familial hypercholesterolaemia. *Neth. J. Med.* 1993 Dec;43(5-6):254-61.

[157] Bredie SJ, de Bruin TW, Demacker PN, Kastelein JJ, Stalenhoef AF. Comparison of gemfibrozil versus simvastatin in familial combined hyperlipidemia and effects on apolipoprotein-B-containing lipoproteins, low-density lipoprotein subfraction profile, and low-density lipoprotein oxidizability. *Am. J. Cardiol.* 1995 Feb 15;75(5):348-53.

[158] Jeck T, Riesen WF, Keller U. Comparison of bezafibrate and simvastatin in the treatment of dyslipidaemia in patients with NIDDM. *Diabet Med.* 1997 Jul;14(7):564-70.

[159] Hoogerbrugge N, Jansen H, De Heide L, Zillikens MC, Deckers JW, Birkenhager JC. The additional effects of acipimox to simvastatin in the treatment of combined hyperlipidaemia. *J. Intern. Med.* 1998 May;243(5):151-6.

[160] Lagrost L, Athias A, Lemort N, Richard JL, Desrumaux C, Chatenet-Duchene L, Courtois M, Farnier M, Jacotot B, Braschi S, Gambert P. Plasma lipoprotein distribution and lipid transfer activities in patients with type IIb hyperlipidemia treated with simvastatin. *Atherosclerosis.* 1999 Apr;143(2):415-25.

[161] Nishikawa O, Mune M, Miyano M, Nishide T, Nishide I, Maeda A, Kimura K, Takahashi T, Kishino M, Tone Y, Otani H, Ogawa A, Maeda T, Yukawa S. Effect of simvastatin on the lipid profile of hemodialysis patients. *Kidney Int. Suppl.* 1999 Jul;71:S219-21.

[162] Geiss HC, Schwandt P, Parhofer KG. Influence of simvastatin on LDL-subtypes in patients with heterozygous familial hypercholesterolemia and in patients with diabetes mellitus and mixed hyperlipoproteinemia. *Exp. Clin. Endocrinol. Diabetes.* 2002 Jun;110(4):182-7.

[163] van den Akker JM, Bredie SJ, Diepenveen SH, van Tits LJ, Stalenhoef AF, van Leusen R. Atorvastatin and simvastatin in patients on hemodialysis: effects on lipoproteins, C-reactive protein and in vivo oxidized LDL. *J. Nephrol.* 2003 Mar-Apr;16(2):238-44.

[164] van Tits LJ, Smilde TJ, van Wissen S, de Graaf J, Kastelein JJ, Stalenhoef AF. Effects of atorvastatin and simvastatin on low-density lipoprotein subfraction profile, low-density lipoprotein oxidizability, and antibodies to oxidized low-density lipoprotein in relation to carotid intima media thickness in familial hypercholesterolemia. *J. Investig. Med.* 2004 Apr;52(3):177-84.

[165] Moriguchi EH, Vieira JL, Itakura H. Differences in the effects of fluvastatin on lipoprotein subclasses distribution is dependent on triglyceride levels. *Atherosclerosis.* 2001; (Suppl. 2):140-141. (abstract)

[166] Marz W, Scharnagl H, Abletshauser C, Hoffmann MM, Berg A, Keul J, Wieland H, Baumstark MW. Fluvastatin lowers atherogenic dense low-density lipoproteins in postmenopausal women with the atherogenic lipoprotein phenotype. *Circulation.* 2001;103(15):1942-8.

[167] Winkler K, Abletshauser C, Hoffmann MM, Friedrich I, Baumstark MW, Wieland H, Marz W. Effect of fluvastatin slow-release on low density lipoprotein (LDL) subfractions in patients with type 2 diabetes mellitus: baseline LDL profile determines specific mode of action. *J. Clin. Endocrinol. Metab.* 2002;87(12):5485-90.

[168] Yoshino G, Hirano T, Kazumi T, Takemoto M, Ohashi N. Fluvastatin increases LDL particle size and reduces oxidative stress in patients with hyperlipidemia. *J. Atheroscler. Thromb.* 2003;10(6):343-7.

[169] Winkler K, Abletshauser C, Friedrich I, Hoffmann MM, Wieland H, Marz W. Fluvastatin slow-release lowers platelet-activating factor acetyl hydrolase activity: a placebo-controlled trial in patients with type 2 diabetes. *J. Clin. Endocrinol. Metab.* 2004;89(3):1153-9.

[170] Shimabukuro M, Higa N, Asahi T, Oshiro Y, Takasu N. Fluvastatin improves endothelial dysfunction in overweight postmenopausal women through small dense low-density lipoprotein reduction. *Metabolism.* 2004;53(6):733-9.

[171] Yuan JN, Tsai MY, Hegland J, Hunninghake DB. Effects of fluvastatin (XU 62-320), an HMG-CoA reductase inhibitor, on the distribution and composition of low density lipoprotein subspecies in humans. *Atherosclerosis.* 1991;87(2-3):147-57.

[172] Superko HR, Krauss RM, DiRicco C. Effect of fluvastatin on low-density lipoprotein peak particle diameter. *Am J Cardiol.* 1997;80(1):78-81.

[173] Hoogerbrugge N, Jansen H. Atorvastatin increases low-density lipoprotein size and enhances high-density lipoprotein cholesterol concentration in male, but not in female patients with familial hypercholesterolemia. *Atherosclerosis.* 1999 Sep;146(1):167-74.

[174] Guerin M, Lassel TS, Le Goff W, Farnier M, Chapman MJ. Action of atorvastatin in combined hyperlipidemia : preferential reduction of cholesteryl ester transfer from HDL to VLDL1 particles. *Arterioscler. Thromb. Vasc. Biol.* 2000 Jan;20(1):189-97.

[175] Nordoy A, Hansen JB, Brox J, Svensson B. Effects of atorvastatin and omega-3 fatty acids on LDL subfractions and postprandial hyperlipemia in patients with combined hyperlipemia. *Nutr. Metab. Cardiovasc. Dis.* 2001 Feb;11(1):7-16.

[176] Freed MI, Ratner R, Marcovina SM, Kreider MM, Biswas N, Cohen BR, Brunzell JD; Rosiglitazone Study 108 investigators. Effects of rosiglitazone alone and in combination with atorvastatin on the metabolic abnormalities in type 2 diabetes mellitus. *Am. J. Cardiol.* 2002 Nov 1;90(9):947-52.

[177] Pontrelli L, Parris W, Adeli K, Cheung RC. Atorvastatin treatment beneficially alters the lipoprotein profile and increases low-density lipoprotein particle diameter in patients with combined dyslipidemia and impaired fasting glucose/type 2 diabetes. *Metabolism.* 2002 Mar;51(3):334-42.

[178] Forster LF, Stewart G, Bedford D, Stewart JP, Rogers E, Shepherd J, Packard CJ, Caslake MJ. Influence of atorvastatin and simvastatin on apolipoprotein B metabolism in moderate combined hyperlipidemic subjects with low VLDL and LDL fractional clearance rates. *Atherosclerosis.* 2002 Sep;164(1):129-45.

[179] Guerin M, Lassel TS, Le Goff W, Farnier M, Chapman MJ. Action of atorvastatin in combined hyperlipidemia : preferential reduction of cholesteryl ester transfer from HDL to VLDL1 particles. *Arterioscler. Thromb. Vasc. Biol.* 2000 Jan;20(1):189-97.

[180] Sasaki S, Kuwahara N, Kunitomo K, Harada S, Yamada T, Azuma A, Takeda K, Nakagawa M. Effects of atorvastatin on oxidized low-density lipoprotein, low-density lipoprotein subfraction distribution, and remnant lipoprotein in patients with mixed hyperlipoproteinemia. *Am. J. Cardiol.* 2002 Feb 15;89(4):386-9.

[181] Tsimihodimos V, Karabina SA, Tambaki AP, Bairaktari E, Goudevenos JA, Chapman MJ, Elisaf M, Tselepis AD. Atorvastatin preferentially reduces LDL-associated platelet-activating factor acetylhydrolase activity in dyslipidemias of type IIA and type IIB. *Arterioscler Thromb Vasc Biol.* 2002 Feb 1;22(2):306-11.

[182] Sakabe K, Fukuda N, Wakayama K, Nada T, Shinohara H, Tamura Y. Effects of atorvastatin therapy on the low-density lipoprotein subfraction, remnant-like particles cholesterol, and oxidized low-density lipoprotein within 2 weeks in hypercholesterolemic patients. *Circ. J.* 2003 Oct;67(10):866-70.

[183] Lariviere M, Lamarche B, Pirro M, Hogue JC, Bergeron J, Gagne C, Couture P. Effects of atorvastatin on electrophoretic characteristics of LDL particles among subjects with heterozygous familial hypercholesterolemia. *Atherosclerosis.* 2003 Mar;167(1):97-104.

[184] Lemieux I, Salomon H, Despres JP. Contribution of apo CIII reduction to the greater effect of 12-week micronized fenofibrate than atorvastatin therapy on triglyceride levels and LDL size in dyslipidemic patients. *Ann. Med.* 2003;35(6):442-8.

[185] Wagner AM, Jorba O, Bonet R, Ordonez-Llanos J, Perez A. Efficacy of atorvastatin and gemfibrozil, alone and in low dose combination, in the treatment of diabetic dyslipidemia. *J. Clin. Endocrinol. Metab.* 2003 Jul;88(7):3212-7.

[186] Brousseau ME, Schaefer EJ, Wolfe ML, Bloedon LT, Digenio AG, Clark RW, Mancuso JP, Rader DJ. Effects of an inhibitor of cholesteryl ester transfer protein on HDL cholesterol. *N. Engl. J. Med.* 2004 Apr 8;350(15):1505-15.

[187] Lins RL, Matthys KE, Billiouw JM, Dratwa M, Dupont P, Lameire NH, Peeters PC, Stolear JC, Tielemans C, Maes B, Verpooten GA, Ducobu J, Carpentier YA. Lipid and apoprotein changes during atorvastatin up-titration in hemodialysis patients with hypercholesterolemia: a placebo-controlled study. *Clin. Nephrol.* 2004 Oct;62(4):287-94.

[188] O'Keefe JH Jr, Captain BK, Jones PG, Harris WS. Atorvastatin reduces remnant lipoproteins and small, dense low-density lipoproteins regardless of the baseline lipid pattern. *Prev. Cardiol.* 2004 Fall;7(4):154-60.

[189] Frost RJ, Otto C, Geiss HC, Schwandt P, Parhofer KG. Effects of atorvastatin versus fenofibrate on lipoprotein profiles, low-density lipoprotein subfraction distribution, and hemorheologic parameters in type 2 diabetes mellitus with mixed hyperlipoproteinemia. *Am. J. Cardiol.* 2001 Jan 1;87(1):44-8.

[190] Geiss HC, Otto C, Schwandt P, Parhofer KG. Effect of atorvastatin on low-density lipoprotein subtypes in patients with different forms of hyperlipoproteinemia and control subjects. *Metabolism.* 2001 Aug;50(8):983-8.

[191] Melenovsky V, Malik J, Wichterle D, Simek J, Pisarikova A, Skrha J, Poledne R, Stavek P, Ceska R. Comparison of the effects of atorvastatin or fenofibrate on nonlipid biochemical risk factors and the LDL particle size in subjects with combined hyperlipidemia. *Am. Heart. J.* 2002 Oct;144(4):E6.

[192] Tsimihodimos V, Karabina SA, Tambaki A, Bairaktari E, Achimastos A, Tselepis A, Elisaf M. Effect of atorvastatin on the concentration, relative distribution, and chemical composition of lipoprotein subfractions in patients with dyslipidemias of type IIA and IIB. *J. Cardiovasc. Pharmacol.* 2003 Aug;42(2):304-10.

[193] Soedamah-Muthu SS, Colhoun HM, Thomason MJ, Betteridge DJ, Durrington PN, Hitman GA, Fuller JH, Julier K, Mackness MI, Neil HA; CARDS Investigators. The effect of atorvastatin on serum lipids, lipoproteins and NMR spectroscopy defined lipoprotein subclasses in type 2 diabetic patients with ischaemic heart disease. *Atherosclerosis.* 2003 Apr;167(2):243-55.

[194] Manuel-Y-Keenoy B, Van Campenhout C, Vertommen J, De Leeuw I. Effects of Atorvastatin on LDL sub-fractions and peroxidation in type 1 diabetic patients: a randomised double-blind placebo-controlled study. *Diabetes Metab. Res. Rev.* 2003 Nov-Dec;19(6):478-86.

[195] van den Akker JM, Bredie SJ, Diepenveen SH, van Tits LJ, Stalenhoef AF, van Leusen R. Atorvastatin and simvastatin in patients on hemodialysis: effects on lipoproteins, C-reactive protein and in vivo oxidized LDL. *J. Nephrol.* 2003 Mar-Apr;16(2):238-44.

[196] Empen K, Geiss HC, Lehrke M, Otto C, Schwandt P, Parhofer KG. Effect of atorvastatin on lipid parameters, LDL subtype distribution, hemorrheological parameters and adhesion molecule concentrations in patients with hypertriglyceridemia. *Nutr. Metab. Cardiovasc. Dis.* 2003 Apr;13(2):87-92.

[197] Ikejiri A, Hirano T, Murayama S, Yoshino G, Gushiken N, Hyodo T, Taira T, Adachi M. Effects of atorvastatin on triglyceride-rich lipoproteins, low-density lipoprotein subclass, and C-reactive protein in hemodialysis patients. *Metabolism.* 2004 Sep;53(9):1113-7.

[198] Dornbrook-Lavender KA, Joy MS, Denu-Ciocca CJ, Chin H, Hogan SL, Pieper JA. Effects of atorvastatin on low-density lipoprotein cholesterol phenotype and C-reactive protein levels in patients undergoing long-term dialysis. *Pharmacotherapy.* 2005 Mar;25(3):335-44.

[199] Caslake MJ, Stewart G, Day SP, Daly E, McTaggart F, Chapman MJ, Durrington P, Laggner P, Mackness M, Pears J, Packard CJ. Phenotype-dependent and -independent actions of rosuvastatin on atherogenic lipoprotein subfractions in hyperlipidaemia. *Atherosclerosis.* 2003;171(2):245-53.

[200] Packard CJ. LDL subfractions and atherogenicity: an hypothesis from the University of Glasgow. *Curr. Med. Res. Opin.* 1996; 13:379-90.

[201] Vakkilainen J, Mero N, Schweizer A, Foley JE, Taskinen MR. Effects of nateglinide and glibenclamide on postprandial lipid and glucose metabolism in type 2 diabetes. *Diabetes Metab. Res. Rev.* 2002; 18:484-90.

[202] Badiou S, Merle De Boever C, Dupuy AM, Baillat V, Cristol JP, Reynes J. Fenofibrate improves the atherogenic lipid profile and enhances LDL resistance to oxidation in HIV-positive adults. *Atherosclerosis.* 2004; 172:273-9.

[203] Tsimihodimos V, Kakafika A, Tambaki AP, Bairaktari E, Chapman MJ, Elisaf M, Tselepis AD. Fenofibrate induces HDL-associated PAF-AH but attenuates enzyme activity associated with apoB-containing lipoproteins. *J. Lipid. Res.* 2003; 44:927-34.

[204] Guerin M, Bruckert E, Dolphin PJ, Turpin G, Chapman MJ. Fenofibrate reduces plasma cholesteryl ester transfer from HDL to VLDL and normalizes the atherogenic, dense LDL profile in combined hyperlipidemia. *Arterioscler. Thromb. Vasc. Biol.* 1996; 16:763-72.

[205] Chapman MJ, Guerin M, Bruckert E. Atherogenic, dense low-density lipoproteins. Pathophysiology and new therapeutic approaches. *Eur. Heart. J.* 1998; 19 Suppl A:A24-30.

[206] Feher MD, Caslake M, Foxton J, Cox A, Packard CJ. Atherogenic lipoprotein phenotype in type 2 diabetes: reversal with micronised fenofibrate. *Diabetes Metab. Res. Rev.* 1999; 15:395-9.

[207] Tan CE, Chew LS, Tai ES, Chio LF, Lim HS, Loh LM, Shepherd J. Benefits of micronised Fenofibrate in type 2 diabetes mellitus subjects with good glycemic control. *Atherosclerosis.* 2001; 154:469-74.

[208] Deighan CJ, Caslake MJ, McConnell M, Boulton-Jones JM, Packard CJ. Comparative effects of cerivastatin and fenofibrate on the atherogenic lipoprotein phenotype in proteinuric renal disease. *J. Am. Soc. Nephrol.* 2001; 12:341-8.

[209] Yuan J, Tsai MY, Hunninghake DB. Changes in composition and distribution of LDL subspecies in hypertriglyceridemic and hypercholesterolemic patients during gemfibrozil therapy. *Atherosclerosis.* 1994 ; 110:1-11.

[210] Yoshida H, Ishikawa T, Ayaori M, Shige H, Ito T, Suzukawa M, Nakamura H. Beneficial effect of gemfibrozil on the chemical composition and oxidative susceptibility of low density lipoprotein: a randomized, double-blind, placebo-controlled study. *Atherosclerosis.* 1998; 139:179-87.

[211] Vakkilainen J, Steiner G, Ansquer JC, Aubin F, Rattier S, Foucher C, Hamsten A, Taskinen MR; DAIS Group. Relationships between low-density lipoprotein particle size, plasma lipoproteins, and progression of coronary artery disease: the Diabetes Atherosclerosis Intervention Study (DAIS). *Circulation.* 2003; 107:1733-7.

[212] Farnier M, Freeman MW, Macdonell G, Perevozskaya I, Davies MJ, Mitchel YB, Gumbiner B; the Ezetimibe Study Group. Efficacy and safety of the coadministration of ezetimibe with fenofibrate in patients with mixed hyperlipidaemia. *Eur. Heart J.* 2005; 26:897-905.

[213] Ikewaki K, Tohyama J, Nakata Y, Wakikawa T, Kido T, Mochizuki S. Fenofibrate effectively reduces remnants, and small dense LDL, and increases HDL particle

number in hypertriglyceridemic men - a nuclear magnetic resonance study. *J. Atheroscler. Thromb.* 2004; 11:278-85.

[214] Ikewaki K, Noma K, Tohyama J, Kido T, Mochizuki S. Effects of bezafibrate on lipoprotein subclasses and inflammatory markers in patients with hypertriglyceridemia--a nuclear magnetic resonance study. *Int. J. Cardiol.* 2005; 101:441-7.

[215] Badiou S, De Boever CM, Dupuy AM, Baillat V, Cristol JP, Reynes J. Small dense LDL and atherogenic lipid profile in HIV-positive adults: influence of lopinavir/ritonavir-containing regimen. *AIDS.* 2003; 17:772-4.

[216] Superko RH, Berneis KK, William PT, Rizzo M, Wood PD. Gemfibrozil reduces small low-density lipoprotein more in normolipemic subjects classified as low-density lipoprotein pattern B compared with pattern A. *Am. J. Card.* 2005. 96(9): 1266-72.

[217] Hokanson JE, Austin MA, Zambon A, Brunzell JD. Plasma triglyceride and LDL heterogeneity in familial combined hyperlipidemia. *Arterioscler. Thromb.* 1993; 13:427-34.

[218] Manninen V, Tenkanen L, Koskinen P, et al. Joint effects of serum triglyceride and LDL cholesterol and HDL cholesterol concentrations on coronary heart disease risk in the Helsinki Heart Study. *Circulation* 1992; 85:37-45.

[219] Tenkanen L, Manttari M, Manninen V. Some coronary risk factors related to the insulin resistance syndrome and the treatment with gemfibrozil. Experience from the Helsinki Heart Study. *Circulation* 1995; 92:1779-1785.

[220] Rubins HB, Robins SJ, Collins D, et al. Gemfibrozil for the secondary prevention of coronary heart disease in men with low levels of high density lipoprotein cholesterol: Veterans Affairs High-density Lipoprotein Cholesterol Intervention Trials Study Group. *N. Engl. J. Med.* 1999; 341:410-418.

[221] Sacks FM, Pfeffer MA, Moye LA, et al. The effect of pravastatin on coronary events after myocardial infarction in patients with average cholesterol levels. *N. Engl. J. Med.* 1996; 335:1001-1009.

[222] The Long-term Intervention with Pravastatin in Ischemic Heart Disease (LIPID) Study Group. Prevention of cardiovascular events and deaths with pravastatin in patients with coronary heart disease and a broad range of initial cholesterol levels. *N. Engl. J. Med.* 1998; 339:1349-1357.

[223] Downs JR, Beere PA, Whitney E, et al. Design and rationale of the Air Force/Texas Coronary Atherosclerosis Prevention Study (AFCAPS/TexCAPS). *Am. J. Cardiol.* 1997; 80:287-293.

[224] Williams PT, Superko HR, Haskell WL, Alderman EA, Blanche PJ, Holl LG, Krauss RM. Smallest LDL particles are most strongly related to coronary disease progression in men. *Arterioscler. Thromb. Vasc. Biol.* 2003;23:314–321.

[225] Miller BD, Alderman EL, Haskell WL, Fair JM, Krauss RM. Predominance of dense low-density lipoprotein particles predicts angiographic benefit of therapy in the Stanford Coronary Risk Intervention Project. *Circulation* 1996; 94:2146–2153

[226] Zambon A, Hokanson JE, Brown BG, Brunzell JD. Evidence for a new pathophysiological mechanism for coronary artery disease regression: hepatic lipase-mediated changes in LDL density. *Circulation* 1999; 99:1959-64.

[227] Rosenson RS, Otvos JD, Freedman DS. Relations of lipoprotein subclass levels and low-density lipoprotein size to progression of coronary artery disease in the Pravastatin Limitation of Atherosclerosis in the Coronary Arteries (PLAC-I) trial. *Am. J. Cardiol.* 2002; 90:89–94

[228] Lamarche B, Lemieux I, Despres JP. The small, dense LDL phenotype and the risk of coronary heart disease: epidemiology, patho-physiology and therapeutic aspects. *Diabetes Metab.* 1999; 25:199-211.

[229] Caslake MJ, Packard CJ. Phenotypes, genotypes and response to statin therapy. Curr *Opin. Lipidol.* 2004; 15:387-92.

[230] Lada AT, Rudel LL. Associations of low density lipoprotein particle composition with atherogenicity. *Curr. Opin. Lipidol.* 2004; 15:19-24.

[231] Marais AD. Therapeutic modulation of low-density lipoprotein size. *Curr. Opin. Lipidol.* 2000; 11:597-602.

[232] Rizzo M, Berneis K, Corrado E, Novo S. The significance of low-density lipoproteins size in vascular diseases. *Int. Angiol.* 2006; 25: 4-9.

[233] Rizzo M, Berneis K. Low-density-lipoproteins size and cardiovascular prevention. *Eur. J. Int. Med.* 2006; 17: 77-80.

[234] Nesto RW. Beyond low-density lipoprotein: addressing the atherogenic lipid triad in type 2 diabetes mellitus and the metabolic syndrome. *Am. J. Cardiovasc. Drugs.* 2005; 5:379-87.

[235] Colhoun HM, Betteridge DJ, Durrington PN, Hitman GA, Neil HA, Livingstone SJ, Thomason MJ, Mackness MI, Charlton-Menys V, Fuller JH; CARDS investigators. Primary prevention of cardiovascular disease with atorvastatin in type 2 diabetes in the Collaborative Atorvastatin Diabetes Study (CARDS): multicentre randomised placebo-controlled trial. *Lancet.* 2004; 364:685-96.

[236] Tenenbaum A, Motro M, Fisman EZ, Tanne D, Boyko V, Behar S. Bezafibrate for the secondary prevention of myocardial infarction in patients with metabolic syndrome. *Arch. Intern. Med.* 2005; 165:1154-60.

[237] Keech A, Simes RJ, Barter P, Best J, Scott R, Taskinen MR, Forder P, Pillai A, Davis T, Glasziou P, Drury P, Kesaniemi YA, Sullivan D, Hunt D, Colman P, d'Emden M, Whiting M, Ehnholm C, Laakso M; FIELD study investigators. Effects of long-term fenofibrate therapy on cardiovascular events in 9795 people with type 2 diabetes mellitus (the FIELD study): randomised controlled trial. *Lancet.* 2005; 366:1849-61.

[238] Grundy SM, Cleeman JI, Merz CNB, Brewer HB, Clark LT, Hunninghake DB et al. for the Coordinating Committee of the National Cholesterol Education Program. Implications of Recent Clinical Trials for the National Cholesterol Education Program Adult Treatment Panel III Guidelines. *Circulation* 2004; 110:227-239.

In: Progress in Metabolic Syndrome Research
Editor: G.T. Ulrig, pp. 39-73

ISBN 1-60021-179-8
© 2006 Nova Science Publishers, Inc.

Chapter II

The Etiology of Obesity-Induced Insulin Resistance

Kyle L. Hoehn[1,], William L. Holland[2],*
Trina A. Knotts[3] and Scott A. Summers[2]

[1]Diabetes and Obesity Program, The Garvan Institute of Medical Research,
Darlinghurst, New South Wales, Australia;
[2]Division of Endocrinology, Diabetes, and Metabolism.
University of Utah School of Medicine, Salt Lake City, UT;
[3]Department of Pediatrics, University of Colorado
Health Sciences Center, Aurora, CO.

Abstract

Insulin is an essential hormone with important roles in glucose homeostasis and anabolic metabolism. Cellular and/or molecular defects in insulin action result in a state of *insulin resistance*, which is an essential feature of the diseases type 2 diabetes and the metabolic syndrome. One of the largest correlations to insulin resistance is obesity; specifically the enlargement of adipose tissue in the abdomen. This correlation is unmistakably obvious today as the twin epidemics of obesity and type 2 diabetes have co-emerged. One of the biggest challenges in the field of diabetes research is to determine how the increase in visceral adiposity leads to impaired insulin action. Recently, two hypothetical mechanisms have transpired: (a) obesity shifts the secretory profile of adipose tissue to favor a reduction in nutrient uptake by creating insulin resistance, and/or (b) overloaded fat cells and the increased caloric intake common in obesity leads to the inappropriate storage of lipids in non-adipose tissues where they antagonize insulin action. This review

---

* Correspondence concerning this article should be addressed to Scott Summers. Division of Endocrinology, Diabetes, and Metabolism, University of Utah School of Medicine, Building 585, Room 110, Salt Lake City, UT 84132, USA. scott.summers@hsc.utah.edu

summarizes recent findings implicating each mechanism, alone or in concert, in the etiology of obesity-induced insulin resistance.

Keywords: Insulin resistance, obesity, adipose tissue, metabolism

A. Introduction

Genetic disposition, caloric intake, age, body composition, and physical inactivity can contribute to adiposity and obesity, which are risk factors for insulin resistance and many related cellular and metabolic abnormalities (i.e. hyperglycemia, dyslipidemia, steatosis, chronic sub-clinical inflammation, intracellular stress, hypertension, and alterations in adipocyte biology and secretions). Individuals with various combinations of these abnormalities are classified as having the metabolic syndrome, and are at an increased risk for developing cardiovascular disease, diabetes, and certain forms of cancer [1,2]. *The Metabolic Syndrome* was formerly called the *insulin resistance syndrome* due to the fact that insensitivity to insulin was deemed to be an essential feature of the condition, and possibly the earliest known defect in the sequelae of the metabolic syndrome. Specifically, insulin resistance predates the diseased state, and the morbidity of this condition depends upon the severity of glucose tolerance and the degree of compensatory hyperinsulinemia. Insulin resistance leads to the impairment of cellular function, which underlies metabolic disease. Consequently, determining the etiology of obesity-induced insulin resistance is a major focus for researchers studying metabolic diseases.

Numerous circulating factors including nutrients, hormones, and cytokines influence the metabolic rheostat controlling whole body insulin sensitivity. Two major prevailing hypotheses have emerged explaining how obesity antagonizes normal insulin action. First, chronic caloric surplus and/or fat cell hypertrophy cause certain cell types within adipose tissue (eg. macrophages and adipocytes) to undergo intrinsic transformations that alter their metabolism and profile of cellular secretions. Specifically, these cells respond to excess nutrients by releasing lipids, hormones, and inflammatory molecules that influence insulin sensitivity in skeletal muscle and liver. Second, obesity reveals a condition in which lipids are diverted from adipose tissue and delivered to tissues in excess of their storage or oxidative capacities. This promotes the formation of certain lipid metabolites in non-adipose tissue that antagonize insulin action, and may contribute to the milieu of metabolic disturbances frequently present in the obese.

B. Brief Overview of Energy Homeostasis

Mammals require a continuous supply of energy for survival. The brain, though accounting for less than 2% of total body weight, has a particularly high fuel demand, accounting for approximately 20% of total energy consumption. Other tissues with high energy needs (e.g. skeletal muscle and the liver) efficiently oxidize both fats and glucose, however the brain relies almost exclusively on glucose and requires a steady supply. Glucose is toxic in high concentrations, therefore the body must maintain constant circulating glucose concentrations within a narrow range (i.e. 4-7mM in humans) by balancing the breakdown and absorption of dietary carbohydrates, proteins, and fats with the production of glucose by the liver and kidneys. To maintain blood glucose levels within this limited range despite feeding and fasting intervals, the body has evolved an efficient metabolic system to mediate glucose clearance/appearance. Elaborate inter-organ communications between the adipose tissue, gut, skeletal muscle, liver, central nervous system, kidneys, vasculature, immune cells, adrenal glands, thyroid, and the pancreas are required to achieve nutrient homeostasis. Specifically, the body adjusts its metabolism in response to nutrient availability to either generate (fasting) or store high energy molecules (feeding).

For metabolically healthy individuals, postprandial carbohydrate, fat, and protein are quickly removed from the bloodstream and synthesized into macromolecules that can easily be reclaimed. Glucose that is not immediately oxidized can be stored as glycogen in the liver, skeletal muscle, kidney, and adipose tissue, or as triglyceride (TG) in the liver and adipose tissue. Fats can be metabolized in skeletal muscle and liver for energy, or can be absorbed by the liver and adipose tissue for packaging/storage. Lastly, amino acids are absorbed by most tissues, where approximately 15% is oxidized and 85% is used for protein synthesis [3].

While fasting, blood glucose concentrations are maintained via the catabolism of stored glycogen in the liver and by the *de novo* synthesis of glucose from glycerol and amino acids in the liver and kidneys, respectively. Skeletal muscle is a major storage depot for glycogen, however it does not contribute glucose to the circulation. With prolonged starvation, whole body glycogen stores become depleted, and many organs are forced to rely largely on fatty acids (liver and muscle) and ketones (brain, muscle, and heart) for energy production.

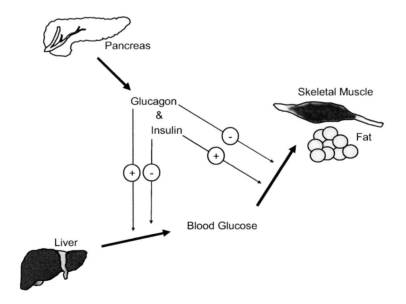

Figure 1. Glucose homeostasis is controlled by the pancreatic hormones insulin and glucagon. Insulin is secreted in response to rising blood glucose concentrations, and has the net effect of reducing blood glucose by inhibiting hepatic glucose production, and stimulating glucose disposal into skeletal muscle and adipose tissues. Glucagon is the catabolic hormone with opposing effects. The body preserves a delicate balance of these two hormones to maintain glucose homeostasis.

C. Insulin Action

The pancreas is a small organ located behind the stomach that has important roles in digestion and metabolism. The endocrine portion of this organ, which exists within the islets of Langerhans, responds to changes in glucose concentrations by secreting insulin or glucagon, two hormones that have opposing actions on glucose homeostasis (Figure 1). While glucagon is a catabolic hormone, insulin is an anabolic one that promotes postprandial nutrient uptake and storage in three major organs: skeletal muscle, liver, and adipose tissue. Specific roles for insulin in regulating glucose, amino acid, and lipid homeostasis in peripheral tissues are briefly discussed here.

C1. Skeletal Muscle

Skeletal muscle tissue is by far the largest consumer of postprandial glucose. Insulin stimulates glucose uptake into this tissue by promoting the translocation of glucose transporter (GluT)-4 containing vesicles to the cell surface where they facilitate diffusion of glucose into the cell. Disparities in translocation vs. transport rates suggests that insulin may additionally activate GluT4; however the mechanisms underlying this effect remain unclear [4,5]. The importance of GluT4 in skeletal muscle is illustrated by mice lacking this protein selectively in this tissue. These animals are glucose intolerant and display hyperglycemia, hyperinsulinemia, and secondary insulin resistance in liver and adipose tissue [6].

In addition to regulating glucose uptake, insulin stimulates various anabolic processes to promote the storage of glucose as glycogen or protein. For example, the hormone increases glycogen storage through inactivation of glycogen synthase kinase (GSK)-3beta and protein kinase A (PKA), which inhibit glycogen synthase (GS), the enzyme which catalyzes the addition of UDP-glucose onto the non-reducing end of existing glycogen strands. Insulin-induced increases in ATP and glucose-6-phosphate concentrations repress rates of glycogen breakdown by inhibiting glycogen phosphorylase, and insulin also simultaneously activates phosphodiesterase (PDE)-3B which hydrolyzes cyclic-AMP and antagonizes PKA activity [7,8]. PKA activates glycogen phosphorylase kinase and inhibits protein phosphatase inhibitor-1; these actions promote phosphorylation and activation of glycogen phosphorylase enzyme and glycogenolysis [9,10]. Insulin increases the rate of protein synthesis by activation of the mammalian target of rapamycin (mTOR)/raptor complex and pp70 S6-kinase pathway, which promotes mRNA translation through eIF4b and decreases protein breakdown by inhibiting lysosomes [11].

C2. Adipose Tissue

In adipocytes, insulin stimulates glucose uptake through GluT4, and promotes glucose storage as both glycogen and lipid. Insulin also promotes fatty acid uptake by stimulating lipoprotein lipase (LPL) activity [12]. LPL converts triglycerides (TG) to free fatty acids (FFA) and glycerol at the plasma membrane, allowing their uptake and re-esterification to

TG. The lipid synthetic enzymes acetyl-CoA carboxylase (ACC) and fatty acid synthase (FAS) are transcriptionally regulated by insulin and synthesize triglycerides *de novo* from acetyl-CoA and glycerol [13,14]. Insulin inhibits lipolysis in adipocytes by signaling the inactivation of the triglyceride lipase hormone sensitive lipase (HSL) [15] through activation of PDE-3B [16,17], which reduces PKA-mediated activation of HSL.

C3. Liver

Glucose uptake in hepatocytes is not regulated in the same manner as in skeletal muscle and adipose tissue. Instead, circulating glucose levels and hepatic expression of glucokinase (GK) play major roles in glucose uptake. Hepatic cells express the high-affinity, insulin-insensitive GluT-2 glucose transporter, which increases glucose uptake into the cell with rising blood glucose in the environment. Insulin plays an indirect role in hepatic glucose uptake by increasing the synthesis of GK enzyme, which converts glucose to glucose-6-phosphate (G6P). G6P is stored as glycogen or metabolized in the pentose phosphate or the glycolytic pathway. The increased rate of glycogen synthesis serves as a driving force for more liver glucose uptake [18].

Insulin stimulates TG production here in a similar mechanism to adipocytes (through FFA absorption and triglyceride synthesis) and inhibits very low density lipoprotein (VLDL)-TG secretion indirectly through its prevention of lipolysis in adipose tissue. Insulin also inhibits hepatic glucose output by blocking gluconeogenesis and glycogenolysis through reduced synthesis of phosphoenolpyruavte carboxykinase (PEPCK) and inactivating glycogen phosphorylase enzyme, respectively [19]. The transcription factors sterol regulatory element binding protein (SREBP)-1c and peroxisome proliferator activated receptor (PPAR)-γ coactivator (PGC)-1α are potentially important mediators of the effect of insulin on hepatic gene expression and metabolism [20,21].

C4. Vasculature, other

Many other cell types express insulin receptors, but their contribution to whole body metabolism is less clear. Insulin stimulates the brain to decrease food intake, the kidney to reduce gluconeogenesis, and reproductive organs to stimulate steroidogenesis. Importantly, insulin action in vascular tissue is important for whole body insulin action and endothelial dysfunction is a major risk factor and early indicator of cardiovascular disease associated with insulin resistance [22]. Endothelial cells make up the lining of blood vessels and secrete various factors that impact vasodilation, vessel tone, and coagulation, etc [23]. These cells are also sensitive to other circulating factors such as angiotensinogen, (a WAT secretagogue whose cleavage product regulates vascular tone) and insulin. Insulin triggers vasodilation by activating endothelial nitric oxide synthase (eNOS), and increasing tetrahydrobiopterin synthesis, an eNOS cofactor [24], in endothelial cells. The activation of vascular nitric oxide production by adiponectin [25,26], the consumption of red wine [27], intake of the dietary flavonoid quercetin [28], or calcium channel blockers [29] offer protective effects from metabolic disease. Additionally, administration of tetrahydrobiopterin partially restores endothelial function in diabetic mice [22].

Quantitatively, this vasodilatory effect may represent an important component of postprandial glucose disposal, as mice with gene disruption of endothelial NOS [30] or both endothelial and neuronal NOS [31] exhibit insulin resistance. In particular, mice lacking eNOS display characteristic features of the metabolic syndrome, including hypertension, dyslipidemia, and insulin resistance [30]. These recent studies in eNOS knockout mice put forth a potential mechanism by which endothelial dysfunction may play a causative, rather than corollary role in metabolic disease. However, the potential mechanism for this hypothesis remains to be discovered.

D. Insulin-Stimulated Signal Transduction

Insulin signaling involves an orderly sequence of ligand binding, protein phosphorylation, and protein-protein interaction events that regulate the synthesis and activity of many molecules important in metabolism and energy expenditure. Herein we concentrate on insulin's regulation of nutrient utilization and disposal, as its effects on cell growth, proliferation, and apoptosis are beyond the scope of this review.

D1. Insulin Receptor

Insulin circulates systemically until it is bound by specific receptor tyrosine kinases (RTKs) exposed on the cell surface. This ligand binding initiates a signal transduction cascade that diverges at multiple downstream effectors. The insulin receptor (IR), insulin receptor-related receptor (IRR), and insulin-like growth factor receptor-1 (IGFR-1) are all tetrameric RTKs composed of two homodimers, each containing an alpha- and beta-subunit. These receptors can heterodimerize to form functional hybrids that maintain various levels of excitability by insulin [32]. Insulin binding to the exposed alpha-subunit reverses its inhibition of the beta-subunits tyrosine kinase activity, leading to activation of the receptor. When stimulated, the receptor will auto-tyrosine phosphorylate itself and regulate at least nine other known proteins by direct phosphorylation and/or interaction.

D2. Insulin Receptor Substrate

Tyrosine phosphorylated RTKs recruit the Insulin Receptor Substrate (IRS) family of proteins. Four mammalian IRS isoforms have been identified, yet only IRS-1 and IRS-2 seem to be important for glucose metabolism [33-35]. Tyrosine phosphorylation of IRS proteins by the IR is stimulatory for IRS function and anabolic signal propagation. However, IRS also has between 30 and 50 potential serine/threonine phosphorylation sites that can either serve to promulgate or inhibit IRS activity depending on the location or possibly the sequence of modification. The phosphorylation status of IRS proteins appears to be a major regulatory mechanism for the efficiency of insulin stimulated signal transduction and for protein stability; they likely play a role in insulin resistance [36].

D3. Phosphatidylinositol-3-kinase (PI3K)

Tyrosyl-phosphorylated IRS proteins recruit and activate the class Ia phosphatidylinositol-3-kinase (PI3K), a lipid kinase composed of a catalytic (p110) subunit, and a regulatory (p85) subunit with two SH2 domains. The SH2 domains of the p85 subunit interact with two tyrosyl-phosphorylated residues on IRS; this induces a conformational change resulting in p110 activation. Once activated, p110 phosphorylates phosphatidylinositides in the plasma membrane at the 3' position resulting in phosphatidylinositol 3,4 bisphosphate (PI(4,5)P2) and phosphatidylinositol 3,4,5 trisphosphate (PI(3,4,5)P3). These phosphorylated lipids then serve to regulate the localization or activity of three main classes of proteins; 1) the cyclic-AMP dependent protein kinase A/ protein kinase G/ protein kinase C (AGC) family of kinases (e.g. Akt/Protein Kinase B, Phosphoinositide Dependent Kinase 1, etc.), 2) the Tec kinases, and 3) the guanine nucleotide exchange factors of Rho GTPases.

D4. Akt/Protein Kinase B, AS160, and GluT4

PI(3,4,5)P3 is a prominent lipid molecule created by insulin-stimulated p110 activity. The presence of PI(3,4,5)P3 in the plasma membrane recruits pleckstrin homology (PH) domain containing proteins to the cell surface. The AGC serine/threonine kinases Phosphoinositide Dependent Kinase-1 (PDK1) and Akt/Protein Kinase B (Akt/PKB) co-localize to the plasma membrane where PDK1 phosphorylates Akt/PKB on a threonine-308 residue in the catalytic domain [37]. Subsequently, an elusive serine 473-kinase phosphorylates Akt/PKB on a serine residue in the c-terminal regulatory motif. The mTOR/Rictor complex appears to be the insulin regulated S473-kinase [38] even though other enzymes can regulate this site in some instances (eg. MAPKAP kinase 2, Akt/PKB, PDK1, ILK, DNA-PK, and PRK2 (reviewed in [39,40])). Either phosphorylation will give partial activity, but both phosphorylations are required for full activation of Akt/PKB.

Akt/PKB is an obligate intermediate in most of insulin's actions [41], including insulin-stimulated glucose uptake via GluT4 externalization, and glycogen synthesis. Akt/PKB is necessary for insulin stimulated glucose uptake; however, its precise contribution in this process is still unknown (see next section). RNA interference studies and knockout mouse models illustrate the importance for Akt2/PKB-beta, but not other (Akt1/PKB-alpha or Akt3/PKBgamma) isoforms in GluT4 trafficking [42,43]. A recent study has shown that a low temperature (19°C) incubation will prevent insulin stimulated Akt/PKB activation and inhibit GluT4 vesicle fusion to the plasma membrane [44]. The low temperature incubation does not inhibit PI3K activity, nor does it prevent the movement of GluT4 vesicles toward the plasma membrane. This suggests the involvement of an Akt/PKB-independent process by which GluT4 vesicles move toward the cell membrane, and an Akt/PKB-dependent event that mediates vesicle docking or fusion with the membrane. Nevertheless, overexpression of constitutively active forms of Akt/PKB [45] or p110 [46] are able to stimulate GluT4 externalization and glucose uptake independent of insulin stimulation.

Mammals have at least 13 different types of GluTs: Class I GluTs (GluTs 1-4) are glucose transporters, Class II GluTs (GluTs 5, 7, 9, and 11) are fructose transporters (a misnomer), and Class III GluTs (GluTs 6, 8, 10, 12 and HMIT-1) are atypical members of this family. Of the Class I GluTs, GluT-1 is ubiquitously expressed and is responsible for basal glucose uptake in most tissues; GluT-2 is found in the β-cells and liver and is important for glucose sensing; GluT-3 is found in brain; and GluT4 is the insulin sensitive glucose transporter found in adipose, cardiac, and skeletal muscle tissue.

GluT4 transporters cycle between the plasma membrane and intracellular compartments at a basal rate. However, upon stimulation by insulin, GluT4 containing vesicles migrate to the cell surface, resulting in increased glucose transport velocity. There are three major steps involved in insulin stimulated glucose transport; translocation and tethering, docking, and vesicle fusion with the membrane. Although it is unknown how insulin-stimulated signaling events converge to drive glucose transport, we do know many of the fundamental steps regulating this process.

Vesicle tethering is facilitated by small Rab GTPases, which bind these vesicles to docking sites on the plasma membrane through the recruitment of other tethering molecules. This is followed by the formation of a stable complex between the vesicle soluble N-ethylmaleimide-sensitive factor attachment protein receptor (v-SNARE) vesicle-associated membrane protein-2 (VAMP-2) containing vesicles (which are enriched in GluT4, and thus also known as GluT4 vesicles) with the target-SNAREs (t-SNAREs) syntaxin-4 and synaptosomal-associated protein (SNAP)-23 at the plasma membrane. This interaction is regulated by Sec1-like/Munc-18 (SM) accessory proteins, which have both positive and negative roles in SNARE complex formation. The last step of GluT4 externalization is vesicle fusion with the membrane. Fusion is facilitated by N-ethylmaleimide sensitive factor (NSF) and SNAP in all SNARE dependent membrane fusions, yet the specific roles of these proteins remain elusive for GluT4 vesicles.

A noteworthy new Akt/PKB substrate, named Akt substrate of 160 kilodaltons (kDa) (AS160), was identified in adipocytes as an important link between Akt/PKB and GluT4 trafficking [47-50]. Insulin stimulation leads to up to five direct phosphorylations of AS160 by Akt/PKB. This phosphorylation is shown to be required for GluT4 translocation and glucose transport. AS160 contains a Rab-GTPase activating protein (Rab-GAP) domain, and is a point of connection linking insulin signaling to Akt/PKB and glucose transport. When active, AS160 keeps Rab proteins in the GDP bound, and inactive form. Upon insulin stimulation, Akt/PKB inactivates AS160 allowing Rab activity and consequently promotes GluT4 vesicle tethering, docking, and fusion. The major hurdle for confirming this hypothesis has been the inability to identify the Rab that AS160 acts upon.

D5. PI3K-Independent Pathway

Recently, an insulin-stimulated PI3-kinase independent pathway has been hypothesized to be compulsory for glucose transport in adipocytes; however, its necessity is currently at the heart of much debate. The proposed pathway results in tyrosine phosphorylation of casitas b-lineage lymphoma (Cbl) by the insulin receptor. Cbl is associated with the adapter protein, Cbl-associated protein (CAP). After the CAP-Cbl complex is phosphorylated, it moves to lipid rafts via CAP interaction with flotillin. The adapter protein CrkII binds phospho-cbl and interacts with the guanine nucleotide exchange factor C3G. Once recruited to the membrane, C3G exchanges GTP for GDP on the G-protein TC10. This exchange activates TC10, which has been described to provide a necessary, but not sufficient, role in GluT4 translocation to the plasma membrane. Several groups have illustrated the necessity of this pathway for GluT4 externalization [51-54], yet others have shown that c-Cbl ablation in mice [55], or the inhibition of this pathway by gene knockdown of CAP, CrkII, and c-Cbl plus Cbl-b, fails to impair glucose transport or GluT4 trafficking [43,56]. Nevertheless, this pathway has been linked to insulin-stimulated recruitment of the exocyst complex and actin assembly, which appear to be important for other processes such as GluT4 recycling [57]. These pathways are summarized in Figure 2.

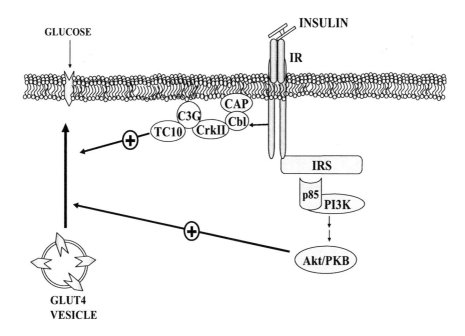

Figure 2. Insulin-stimulated glucose uptake is mediated by the translocation and fusion of GluT4 containing vesicles to the plasma membrane. The precise mechanisms leading to GluT4 externalization remain elusive; however two known pathways that mediate insulin's actions are summarized here.

E. Insulin Resistance and the Metabolic Syndrome

Insulin resistance is the inability to adequately control glucose homeostasis in response to physiologically 'normal' concentrations of insulin. This condition causes decreased glucose uptake and utilization in skeletal muscle, and defective suppression of glucose output from the liver. Interestingly, other insulin-stimulated metabolic events, such as anti-lipolysis and certain mitogenic effects, do not appear to be affected by the insulin resistant state. In early stages of insulin resistance, a compensatory increase in insulin output from the pancreas effectively maintains glucose homeostasis. In some individuals, this compensatory hyperinsulinemia is sufficient to maintain euglycemia, and patients may remain asymptomatic for years or indefinitely. In fact, only approximately one-third of obese individuals fail to maintain this hyperinsulinemia, and ultimately become glucose intolerant or diabetic [58]. However, chronic hyperinsulinemia can be a pathogenic condition in itself, and may precipitate other clinical pathologies [59,60].

The metabolic syndrome is clinically defined as the concurrent presentation of 3 of the following 5 features: waist circumference ≥40 inches in men and ≥35 inches in women; triglycerides level ≥1.70 mM, or person is receiving drug treatment for an elevated level of triglycerides; high-density lipoprotein cholesterol (HDL-C) level <1.04 mM in men and <1.30 mM in women, or person is receiving drug treatment for reduced HDL-C level; blood pressure ≥130 mm Hg (systolic) or ≥85 mm Hg (diastolic), or person is receiving drug treatment for hypertension; elevated fasting glucose level ≥5.55 mM, or person is receiving drug treatment for elevated glucose level [61]. Persons diagnosed with the metabolic syndrome are at a several-fold elevated risk for diabetes, cardiovascular disease, and stroke.

F. The Link between Obesity and Insulin Resistance

Adipose tissue from obese insulin-resistant patients is characterized by hypertrophic fat cells that have altered adipokine secretions and are resistant to insulin-stimulated glucose uptake and suppression of free fatty acid release. Two hypotheses have emerged to explain the link between an individual's degree of adiposity and their state of insulin (in)sensitivity. As aforementioned, adiposity is associated with two factors that render cells insensitive to insulin action; specifically, altered adipokine secretions, and the accumulation of lipids and specific lipid metabolites in non-adipose cells. Importantly, non-overweight individuals with either of these conditions (i.e. chronic inflammation or peripheral steatosis) have increased frequency of insulin resistance [62]. We propose that both mechanisms, either independently or in concert, are involved in the etiology of obesity-induced insulin resistance.

Studies aimed at elucidating a link between increased adiposity and peripheral insulin resistance has led to the new appreciation that white adipose tissue (WAT) is a highly dynamic metabolic and endocrine organ. WAT depots are composed of white adipocytes and stromal/vascular cells, with 11% of the latter being bone marrow derived CD14+/CD31+ macrophages capable of eliciting systemic immune responses [63]. Interestingly, adipocytes themselves also appear to secrete cytokines, chemokines, and hormones that have dual responsibilities in regulating metabolism and inflammation at the whole body level. The precise mechanisms of nutrient sensing remain to be fully understood, however it is known that fat secretagogues act as ligands, second messengers, and transcriptional co-factors that regulate metabolic pathways and gene expression through autocrine, paracrine, and endocrine mechanisms.

WAT secretions are regulated both intrinsically by fat cell hypertrophy, and extrinsically by nutrients, hormones, and inflammatory molecules. With obesity, adipocytes swell in diameter and alter their secretions to favor the repression of food intake and reduction in adipocyte size [64,65]. Specifically, leptin is an adipocyte-derived hormone (adipokine) that signals satiety [66], while free fatty acids [67], TNFα [68], and other signals retard nutrient storage via the inhibition of insulin action. In addition to these secretagogues, the fat cell secretes other insulin-sensitizing adipokines (eg. adiponectin, visfatin, and vaspin) and insulin-desensitizing adipokines (eg. interleukin (IL)-6, retinol binding protein (RBP)-4, plasminogen activator inhibitor (PAI)-1, and resistin) that control fuel homeostasis and insulin action by signaling to the hypothalamus and directly acting on peripheral tissues such as skeletal muscle and the liver. The specific role of each adipokine in insulin action is discussed in detail later in this chapter.

Interestingly, not all obese individuals are insulin resistant, nor are all insulin resistant individuals obese. This condition can occur in normal-weight individuals that have lipid storage defects and/or chronic inflammatory conditions [62]. Conversely, some significantly obese individuals with low ectopic fat accumulation are metabolically normal [69]. Thus, we argue that elevated adiposity is a relative factor that does not directly cause insulin resistance, but rather increases the likelihood of developing the dual threat of ectopic lipid accumulation and chronic inflammation (Figure 3).

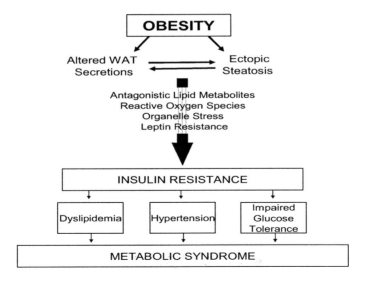

Figure 3. Obesity alters adipose tissue biology in a way that changes its ratio of secretions and sponsors fat accumulation in peripheral tissues. Either of these two means can facilitate the other; however each can antagonize insulin action independently. The development of insulin resistance is a significant risk factor for the progression of metabolic disease.

F1. Abdominal Adiposity

Fat is not distributed evenly across the human body, and the location of adipose stores depends upon a number of variables. Principally there are android-type (apple shaped) and gynoid-type (pear shaped) patterns of fat distribution. Insulin resistance is more closely related to the central or android-type obesity, where fat is preferentially stored in the abdominal region. Subsequently, researchers have begun investigating potential mechanisms for this observation.

Abdominal adipose tissue is comprised of both subcutaneous and intraabdominal depots. Intraabdominal adipose tissue is localized into intraperitoneal and retroperitoneal spaces, with the former also known as visceral adipose tissue (VAT). VAT can then be sub-classified into omental and mesnchymal depots. Subcutaneous adipose tissue (SCAT) in the abdomen is divided into 2 layers by fascia; the outer layer is superficial subcutaneous (SSCAT), and the inner layer is deep subcutaneous (DSCAT). While total abdominal body fat is highly associated with insulin resistance, researchers have performed careful analyses into the specific depots to determine how each may affect insulin sensitivity.

F1a. Fat Depot Characteristics: VAT vs. SCAT

SCAT and VAT demonstrate significant differences that may provide clues regarding their differential roles in the development of insulin resistance. Specifically, the two depots secrete adipokines to differing degrees, demonstrate dissimilar capacities to mobilize FFAs (i.e. VAT is more lipolytically active especially in obesity-induced insulin resistance -- possibly due to reduced PDE-3B levels [70]), and have different proximities to insulin-sensitive organs (i.e. VAT secretions are delivered directly into the portal vein) which may affect liver fat storage or glucose efflux. Specifically, Smith, et al. reported that the size of VAT and DSAT depots (analyzed by CT and DEXA scanning) appear to be more closely associated with increased fasting insulin and triglyceride levels than other fat depots [71]. A number of similar studies evaluated insulin sensitivity in obese volunteers by euglycemic-hyperinsulinemic clamp, a much more accurate determination of insulin action. These studies are reviewed in [72], but failed to come to a consensus regarding depot specific pathogenicity. Although failing to agree on which specific depot is more antagonistic to insulin-stimulated glucose disposal, these studies do agree that insulin-mediated suppression of hepatic glucose production is inversely correlated with both VAT and SCAT.

Recently, a critical VAT threshold (CVATT) hypothesis has been proposed which heavily relies on the hypothesis that VAT is more pathogenic to insulin sensitivity than SCAT. This hypothesis proposes that a threshold exists where once an individual reaches their critical VAT mass they rapidly develop insulin resistance and metabolic dysfunction [73]. Some evidence for the CVATT hypothesis is that the metabolic profiles of patients with visceral obesity are greatly improved with subtle weight loss [74], which is shown to decrease VAT depot first compared to SCAT [75-77]. Secondly, SCAT is believed to serve as a protective lipid sink for the overloaded VAT [78], thus offering protection from insulin resistance. Finally, patients lacking normal amounts of peripheral SCAT due to congenital generalized lipoatrophy or highly active anti-retroviral therapy treatment for HIV are increasingly prone to severe insulin resistance [79-81]. To illustrate the importance of SCAT in insulin action, the transplantation of either visceral or subcutaneous fat from donor animals into the subcutaneous space of lipoatrophic mice results in a reversal of their insulin resistance [82]. Further evidence provided in this hypothesis is that women, who naturally have less visceral fat than men, usually only develop metabolic abnormalities when they have become post-menopausal and accumulate VAT depots equivalent to men [83,84].

Site specific removal of SCAT vs. VAT depots have a varying impact on insulin sensitivity. Hamsters with selective removal of SCAT develop adverse metabolic syndromes [85], while the removal of VAT (epididymal and perinephric fat pads), but not SCAT, in rats reverses hepatic insulin resistance [86]. SCAT removal studies in humans are conflicting, but have been reported to provide beneficial effects on insulin sensitivity. The largest study followed 123 obese women undergoing large volume liposuction and demonstrated that the procedure significantly improved their insulin sensitivity, basal metabolic rate, serum adipocytokine, and inflammatory marker levels within weeks, and the phenotype persisted through the 90 days of the study [87]. Another study of patients undergoing bariatric surgery showed that site specific removal of omental VAT pads in conjunction with the surgery resulted in significantly improved metabolic and inflammatory profiles than did bariatric surgery alone [88]. However, there are some disparities reported from other studies evaluating the effects of liposuction, which may relate to the location of SCAT removal (i.e. from the abdomen versus the arms) [88-91].

The proportion of adipose tissue secretagogues that are released from the two depots also varies for some adipokines. Particularly important is leptin, an insulin-sensitizing adipokine that is secreted at higher levels by SCAT than VAT in humans. Circulating leptin levels therefore depend upon body fat distribution [92] (i.e. an individual with a higher percentage of VAT will have lower leptin levels and presumably less protection from insulin resistance than a person of the same adiposity with a higher percentage of SCAT). This 'relative hypoleptinemia' of individuals with more VAT is another potential mechanism by which VAT may be more pathogenic than SCAT [93]. The roles of leptin and other adipokines in the regulation of insulin action are reviewed in detail later in this chapter.

F1b. Counter-arguments for the Pathogenesis of VAT

There are arguments against visceral fat being involved in insulin resistance. First, the observed high rates of lipolysis in VAT should lead to the disappearance of this depot and amelioration of insulin resistance by itself unless it is matched by high rates of fat deposition, for which there is far less evidence [94]. Second, the proportion of fatty acids in the portal vein that are derived from lipolysis of visceral fat is five times less than the proportion derived from subcutaneous fat in obese persons [72,95]. Third, studies evaluating epididymal VAT accumulation or removal in rodents do not support the hypothesis that accessibility to the portal vein is important for the pathogenesis of insulin resistance. Visceral adipose depots in rodents are composed of mesenteric, retroperitoneal, and epididymal stores; removal of the epididymal depot reverses hepatic insulin resistance, despite the fact that this depot does not drain to the portal vein [86].

Visceral fat is also probably not a major factor in the pathogenesis of intramyocellular lipid (IMCL) accumulation, as it likely only contributes a small percentage of the FFAs that reach skeletal muscle tissue [72,95]. Specifically, in lean vs. obese individuals, the free fatty acids in arterial circulation (which may be utilized by muscle beds) are contributed by upper body SCAT (78% vs. 60%), lower body SCAT (16% vs. 26%), and the liver (including input from the digestive system and VAT) (8% vs. 14%). Overall, this means that VAT contributes only a fraction of the FFAs (0.4% in lean people vs. 2.8% in obese people) that make it through the liver (assuming that 100% of VAT secretions go through portal circulation). Therefore, few fatty acids released from visceral fat ever make it to skeletal muscle [72].

F2. Impaired Glucose Uptake within Fat

Insulin stimulates glucose entry in WAT, and this tissue can also become insulin resistant in the obese. VAT is the more insulin-responsive depot, as it has higher GluT4 levels and twice the rate of insulin stimulated glucose uptake when compared to SCAT [96]. The relative amount of GluT4 is a very important factor, as higher amounts of this transporter may be why triglycerides are preferably stored in VAT, and why adipocytes in this depot become larger and more metabolically active.

Glucose uptake in WAT is not particularly important from the standpoint of reducing glucose levels in the blood; however, WAT glucose uptake has been shown to be important for maintaining whole body insulin sensitivity. Specifically, researchers have recently discovered that GluT4 levels are significantly reduced in obese and insulin resistant humans and rodents [97]. Subsequently her group demonstrated that mice lacking GluT4 in WAT are hyperglycemic and exhibit insulin resistance in liver and muscle tissue [6]. Additionally, when this group made mice overexpressing the GluT4 transgene in fat they discovered that the animals had enhanced glucose utilization and larger epididymal fat pads, but no changes in fat cell size or insulin sensitivity [98].

To identify differentially regulated genes between the transgenic and knockout mice, they performed affymetrix screening on their adipose depots. One of the targets identified was retinol binding protein (RBP)-4, a secretagogue whose biological relevance to insulin action is still unknown. The presence of RBP-4 in circulation is directly correlated with insulin resistance in humans and mice and it appears to be a potential link between GLUT4, WAT, and insulin sensitivity in peripheral tissues [99]. Thus, although WAT doesn't contribute much to the control of blood glucose levels through direct glucose uptake, it has a potentially greater role in controlling blood sugar levels by regulating the secretion of molecules that influence skeletal muscle and liver glucose uptake.

F3. Glucocorticoids

Glucocorticoids regulate protein, fat, and carbohydrate metabolism and influence insulin sensitivity. Though circulating glucocorticoid levels are not elevated in the obese, recent studies suggest that the glucocorticoids synthesized within adipose tissue may account for some of the metabolic disturbances in the insulin resistant obese.

The interconversion of the inactive glucocorticoid cortisone into the active steroid cortisol is performed by the bidirectional enzyme 11-β Hydroxysteroid dehydrogenase type 1

(11-β HSD1). VAT tissue is particularly enriched in both 11beta-HSD1 [100] and glucocorticoid receptors [101]. In mice, the overexpression of 11-β HSD1 in adipose tissue leads to increased adipose levels of corticosterone, and the mice develop visceral obesity, insulin-resistant diabetes, and hyperlipidemia [102]. Interestingly, overexpression of this enzyme selectively in the liver of mice does not induce significant obesity, but leads to lipid accumulation in the liver and development of the metabolic syndrome [103]. The pharmacologic inhibition of 11ß-HSD1 ameliorates high-fat diet induced metabolic abnormalities in mice [104], and the overexpression of 11ß-HSD2, which reduces glucocorticoid activation in adipose tissue, reduces fat accumulation in animals on a high fat diet [105].

F4. Chronic Inflammation with Obesity

Adipose tissue contains fat cells, preadipocytes, endothelial cells, and immune cells. In obese individuals and rodents, there is a significant enrichment of macrophages that infiltrate the fat pad. Recently, researchers have speculated that excess secretion of TNFα by enlarged adipocytes promotes endothelial cell activation and secretion of macrophage chemoattractant protein (MCP)-1, leading to macrophage invasion and activation [106]. One alternate hypothesis is that macrophages are recruited to fat tissue to scavenge the residual lipids from dead fat cells. The macrophages fuse to form activated multinucleate giant cells that secrete inflammatory cytokines [107]. Regardless, of the mechanism, the macrophages amplify the weak inflammatory signals produced by adipocytes, ultimately leading to the development of a chronic sub-clinical inflammatory state.

Chronic low-grade inflammation causes insulin resistance even in the absence of obesity [108,109]. This suggests that macrophage infiltration of adipose tissue may be a cause of insulin resistance rather than a consequence of the condition. Inflammatory cytokines produced within WAT that are highly associated with obesity include TNFα, leptin, and interleukins (IL), etc, and the circulating levels of these WAT-derived secretagogues correlate with obesity and insulin resistance. Moreover, knockout animals lacking important signaling mediators of inflammation-induced insulin resistance (e.g. TNFα or TNFα-receptors, Inhibitor of κB Kinase (IκKβ) and Jun N-terminal Kinase (JNK)) are resistant to obesity-induced insulin resistance [110-113].

F5. The Role of Adipokines in Metabolism, Inflammation, and Insulin Action

Adipokines are low molecular weight peptide hormones derived from white adipose depots. These molecules act upon multiple organs including the brain, liver, skeletal muscle, pancreas, and vasculature to influence energy expenditure and metabolism in an endocrine, paracrine, and autocrine manner. The major adipokines that influence insulin action, and have a possible role in the etiology of insulin resistance are described here.

F5a. Insulin Desensitizing Adipokines: TNF-alpha, IL6, PAI, and Resistin

F5ai. TNFα

TNFα is a pro-inflammatory molecule produced in white adipocyte, macrophage, and skeletal muscle cells. The cytokine is a purported antagonist of insulin action which signals through autocrine and paracrine mechanisms to antagonize insulin signaling and promote lipolysis within WAT. In addition, TNFα may directly regulate insulin action in peripheral tissues, such as skeletal muscle and the liver. Unlike many other adipokines, TNFα is secreted equally by different WAT depots [114]. TNFα converting enzyme (TACE) catalyzes cleavage of a TNFα trimer, releasing a soluble 17kDa form into the circulation. The uncleaved and the soluble form of TNFα retain a variable ability to interact with the two classes of TNFα receptors (TNFRs) present in fat and peripheral tissues [115].

TNFα is regarded as an important contributor to obesity-induced insulin resistance [68,116-119]: (a) the administration of TNFα to otherwise healthy rats [120] or humans [121] will generate insulin resistance; (b) genetically obese insulin resistant animals [122] and centrally obese insulin resistant humans demonstrate elevated levels of TNFα [123,124]; and (c) TNFα or TNFR knockout mice exhibit improved insulin sensitivity with lower levels of circulating free fatty acids, even when made obese [112,125,126].

TNFα induces insulin resistance in skeletal muscle and the liver through several distinct mechanisms. For one, it increases lipolysis within WAT by stimulating HSL expression [128], and thus increases the delivery of FFAs to peripheral tissues. Moreover, it downregulates expression of GluT4 [129] and inhibits insulin signaling at the level of the IR and IRS. The serine/threonine kinases JNK, inhibitor of NF-κB kinase (IKK), and PKC-θ are likely intermediates linking TNFα to the regulation of insulin signaling. These enzymes may directly phosphorylate and inactivate IR and IRS proteins, but also induce changes in gene expression through c-Jun and NFkB. In particular, these transcription factors alter the expression of genes that regulate insulin signaling. One such protein whose expression is regulated by TNFα is suppressor of cytokine signaling (SOCS)-3, a protein that interacts with the IR (and leptin receptor) to block downstream signaling [130]. Lastly, the sphingolipid ceramide is another potential mediator linking TNFα to the inhibition of insulin signaling [131-133]. TNFα stimulates ceramide accumulation by initiating a program for de novo ceramide synthesis and by activating sphingomyelinases (SMases) [134]. Ceramide is also a purported antagonist of both IRS-1 and Akt/PKB (see section F6bii below).

Unfortunately, despite the success of TNFα neutralization in the reversal of insulin resistance in obese rodents, the same treatment in obese human type 2 diabetics showed no benefits [127]. The increased risk of opportunistic infections also makes TNFα neutralization a less popular solution for treatment of insulin resistance. Nevertheless, studies on TNFα have been pioneering, and were critical for identifying WAT as an endocrine organ and for identifying the relationship between obesity and inflammation.

F5aii. IL6

TNFα influences the expression of several other cytokines, including IL6 [135], which is secreted more from visceral than subcutaneous adipose tissue [136]. Adipocytes contribute about 30-50% of IL6 to circulation, while the rest derives from WAT macrophages [137-

139]. Despite the direct correlation with insulin resistance and association with TNFα, less is known about what role IL6 plays in the insulin resistant state. In cultured 3T3-L1 cells [135] and HepG2 hepatocytes [140], IL6 antagonizes insulin action via a SOCS-3 dependent mechanism. Young mice lacking IL6 are leaner than control mice early in age, but they develop obesity and impaired glucose tolerance with time [141,142]. IL6 is produced in significant quantities by muscle beds during exercise, but not at rest, and likely plays an unknown role in sensing energy expenditure.

F5aiii. PAI-1

Plasminogen activator inhibitor-1 (PAI-1) is an inhibitor of tissue-type plasminogen activator, which impairs fibrin degradation and increases thrombosis leading to vascular injuries. Both of these defects are common in individuals with chronic insulin resistance or type 2 diabetes [143]. PAI-1 levels increase in proportion with central obesity, but continue to increase throughout the progression of type 2 diabetes, indicating a possible causal relationship [144,145]. Studies in PAI-1 knockout animals or 3T3-L1 adipocytes incubated with PAI-1 neutralizing antibodies show that the absence or inhibition of PAI-1 promotes glucose uptake and adipocyte differentiation, and protects against insulin resistance [145,146].

F5aiv. Resistin

Resistin is another adipokine secreted from white adipose tissue in direct correlation with obesity [147] with a possible role in insulin resistance [148,149]. In mice, resistin is secreted largely from adipocytes, while in humans it derives from macrophages [150,151]. The administration of recombinant resistin to mice, cultured adipocytes, and cultured myotubes impairs insulin action [147,152]. Moreover, the neutralization of resistin with an anti-resistin antibody protects mice from insulin resistance induced by a high fat diet [147,152].

Studies in cultured L6 rat skeletal muscle cells identified a possible mechanism for resistin's antagonism of insulin signaling. Researchers found that incubating these cells with recombinant resistin reduced the total protein levels of IRS-1 and Akt1, and decreased insulin-stimulated glucose uptake and glycogen synthesis [152]. The relationship between resistin and insulin resistance remains controversial largely because of the lack of an association of resistin levels with insulin resistance in humans [148,153-155]. Interestingly, a recent study proposed that resistin may be a secondary effect of insulin resistance that is secreted in response to chronic inflammation; this group has also speculated that resistin may possibly possess anti-oxidant properties [156].

F5b. Insulin Sensitizing Adipokines: Leptin and Adiponectin

Leptin and adiponectin are adipokines with positive effects on energy expenditure and insulin action. While the full complement of physiological effects of either hormone are yet to be elucidated, studies suggest that they generally improve insulin sensitivity, in part by stimulating fatty-acid oxidation in lean tissues.

F5bi. Leptin

Leptin was originally identified through parabiosis experiments as an absent circulating factor in mouse models of obesity, and the deficiency of the hormone or its receptor (db/db) leads to increased food intake, massive obesity, and insulin resistance [157]. Subsequent studies demonstrating that leptin administration in rodents decreases caloric intake and reduces body weight [158] generated considerable excitement regarding its potential usefulness in negating obesity in humans. However, though leptin has dramatic effects on body habitus and insulin resistance in leptin deficient patients [159] and lipoatrophic diabetics [160], treatment with the adipokine has little effects in common obesity in humans [161].

In addition to having clear roles in the regulation of appetite in rodents, numerous studies show that this adipokine has multiple other roles in the maintenance of energy homeostasis. Of particular note, leptin has been reported to promote oxidation and decrease the storage of lipids, which it achieves by repressing SREBP-1c in liver, pancreas, and adipose tissue [162], and by inhibiting acetyl-CoA carboxylase (ACC) [162,163]. This in turn augments insulin action in muscle and the liver (reviewed in [164]). Since circulating leptin levels are highly correlated with obesity and fat cell size [165], researchers have speculated that the body becomes leptin resistant, which contributes to the overall decrease in insulin sensitivity. This same group has made substantial contributions indicating that leptin resistance is a major metabolic defect that contributes to lipotoxicity and the development of insulin resistance (reviewed in [93]). They propose that the increase in leptin, concomitant with obesity, is in fact a side effect of leptin resistance. The rise in leptin thus protects non-adipose tissues from further lipid accumulation. Supporting this, transgenic mice overexpressing leptin receptors selectively in adipose tissue were protected from leptin resistance, adipocyte hypertrophy and hyperplasia, and increased body fat resulting from high fat feeding [166]. Interestingly, overexpression of leptin receptor-b explicitly in neurons fully normalizes the obesity, diabetes, and infertility phenotypes of db/db mice that lack this gene [167].

SH2-containing protein tyrosine phosphatase (SHP)-2, SOCS-3, or protein tyrosine phosphatase (PTP)-1B all negatively regulate the leptin receptor, and each has been implicated as a putative intermediate accounting for leptin resistance [168-171]. A recent study revealed that high-fat feeding for a mere six days induced leptin resistance through a 22-fold increase in SOCS-3 protein in WAT, and a subsequent decrease in leptin receptor-b mRNA. Although not clearly associated with obesity, another possible mechanism for leptin resistance is the cleavage of the leptin receptor at the extracellular surface, creating a soluble moiety that can modulate leptin action [172,173].

F5bii. Adiponectin

Adiponectin is a WAT-derived hormone with a secretion profile that inversely correlates with adiposity [174]. The decrease in adiponectin levels may be a secondary effect caused by an increase in TNFα and IL6, both of which antagonize adiponectin production [175]. Adiponectin exists in diverse molecular states including monomers, trimers, hexamers (180 kDa, low molecular weight), and multimers of up to 18 units (400-540 kDa, high molecular weight) [179]. The higher molecular weight complexes have the greatest correlation with glucose tolerance in humans, and thus appear to be the bioactive forms

[180]. However, deletion of the collagenase domain of this protein and overexpression in rodents increases lipid clearance while enhancing insulin action, despite its inability to form multimeric complexes [177].

Studies in isolated cells or tissues indicate that adiponectin, by activating AMP-activated protein kinase (AMPK), promotes fatty acid oxidation and glucose uptake while inhibiting hepatic glucose production. Animal models showing alterations in adiponectin support a role for the importance of this hormone in the regulation of insulin sensitivity and nutrient disposal. First, mice lacking adiponectin develop very severe insulin resistance when fed a high fat diet [176]. Second, overexpression of an adiponectin construct lacking its collagenase domain leads to a 3-fold increase in circulating adiponectin levels and improved lipid clearance and insulin action [177]. And third, administration of recombinant adiponectin protects leptin deficient mice from insulin resistance and diabetes [178]. Thus, the absence of adiponectin may be an underlying cause of insulin resistance.

Adiponectin's capacity to prevent lipid accumulation in non-adipose tissue, coupled with its anti-inflammatory and cardioprotective effects may prove to be a beneficial therapy for obesity and its related complications. Adiponectin increases expression of anti-inflammatory cytokines IL-10 and IL-1 receptor antagonist in macrophages, inhibits IL6 and TNFα expression, and blocks the activity of TNFα. Another benefit of adiponectin is that it downregulates the expression of adhesion molecules in endothelial cells, which protects against macrophage infiltration into adipose tissue. Treatment with adiponectin therefore protects against the dangers of both inflammation and ectopic lipid accumulation, and promises an exciting prospective therapy for improving metabolic function.

F6. Aberrant Lipid Accumulation as an Underlying Cause of Insulin Resistance

When regarding the mechanisms linking obesity to insulin resistance, perhaps the greatest insight derives from studies on normal weight individuals who demonstrate metabolic dysfunction. Some individuals with normal body mass indexes have metabolic abnormalities typically present in the obese. For example, patients with hypertriglyceridemia, increased PAI-1 levels, post-myocardial infarction, polycystic ovary disease, gout, hypertension, non-alcoholic fatty liver disease (NAFLD), rheumatoid arthritis, hepatitis and some forms of cancer are susceptible to insulin resistance in the absence of obesity [62,181-185]. Moreover, people with low levels of subcutaneous fat due to genetic lipoatropy or advanced anti-retroviral therapy for HIV also exhibit metabolic defects in insulin action [186,187].

Animal models also exist where insulin resistance is present in the absence of obesity. First, the adipose-specific overexpression of diacylglycerol aclytransferase-1 (Dgat1) in mice leads to diet-induced insulin resistance in the absence of obesity or the redistribution of fat from adipose tissue to the liver. This mechanism appears to occur through an upregulation in the gluconeogenic enzymes glucose-6-phosphatase and PEPCK [188]. Another model (as previously mentioned) illustrated that overexpression of the 11ß-HSD1 enzyme selectively in liver did not induce obesity, yet promoted lipid accumulation in the liver and caused insulin resistance [103]. The commonality between most of these conditions is that dyslipidemia and/or elevated circulating lipid levels are still present even in the absence of obesity.

F6a. Accumulation of Lipids in Lean Tissues

Using nuclear magnetic resonance techniques researchers recently determined that intramyocellular lipid levels correlated more tightly with the severity of insulin resistance than other known risk factors including body mass index (BMI), percent body fat, waist-to-hip ratio, or age [69,189]. These observations have fueled the hypothesis that insulin resistance results from the aberrant deposition of lipids in peripheral tissues.

In healthy individuals, fats are stored largely in white adipose tissue (WAT) depots, and the rates of lipolysis are tightly controlled by insulin. In stark opposition, lipolysis goes unchecked in diabetic animals resulting in severe elevations in triglyceride and free fatty acids. Interestingly, the effective concentration (EC50) of insulin required for suppression of lipolysis in adipose tissue falls between 7-16 μU/ml, well below the physiological concentration required for other insulin-stimulated events [190]. Thus, in mildly insulin resistant states, insulin would likely still prevent lipolysis, but may increase blood lipid levels by not stimulating lipogenesis in adipose tissue. With continued over-nutrition there is further development of obesity and more severe insulin resistance. As such, this EC50 value increases 2 to 3-fold, making insulin less effective at repressing lipolysis [190]. Thus, when in a fully insulin resistant state the subnormal suppression of lipolysis, and decreased lipogenesis in adipose tissue might promote hyperlipidemia and the diversion of lipid into less suitable tissues such as muscle and liver.

While it is clear that severe insulin resistance will induce aberrant lipid accumulation in skeletal muscle and the liver, and that lipid accumulation will exacerbate the insulin resistant state, it is less clear whether this aberrant lipid disposal can is a primary event in the development of insulin resistance. Specifically, is the tight correlation between IMCL levels and insulin resistance simply because IMCL is a relatively sensitive indicator of insulin resistance? Interestingly, several studies suggest that experimental manipulations designed to promote lipid storage in skeletal muscle or the liver are sufficient to induce insulin resistance. For example, infusing lipids directly into the bloodstream of rats, mice, or humans is sufficient to antagonize insulin action [191]. Second, overexpressing lipoprotein lipase in skeletal muscle or liver of transgenic mice compromises insulin-stimulated glucose uptake [192,193]. A question remaining is whether preventing lipid accumulation or metabolism in these peripheral tissues is sufficient to ameliorate insulin resistance. Regardless, these findings suggest that excessive lipid deposition in peripheral tissues may be a primary cause, and not merely a consequence, of insulin resistance.

F6b. Mechanisms of Lipid-Induced Insulin Resistance

The mechanisms by which excess lipid down-regulates insulin action is unclear, and multiple pathways may link exogenous fats to the development of insulin resistance. A relationship through which excess fats block glucose oxidation, and ultimately glucose uptake, was described in 1963 by Randle and coworkers [194]. This "Randle Hypothesis" is that glucose and lipids serve as competitive substrates for oxidation, and that increased FFA flux would elevate acetyl-CoA levels, thus decreasing pyruvate dehydrogenase activity and increasing cytosolic citrate. This increase in intracellular citrate would ultimately decrease glycolysis and inhibit glucose phosphorylation and uptake [194].

While the Randle hypothesis likely contributes to impairments in glucose utilization, subsequent studies revealed that defects in insulin signal transduction may serve as primary events in the regulation of glucose utilization [67,195-197]. Researchers have since hypothesized that specific fat-derived metabolites, such as ceramide, fatty acyl-CoA and diacylglycerol (DAG), mediate this effect by initiating pathways leading to the inactivation of insulin signaling intermediates.

F6bi. Diacylglycerol

Many groups have proposed that DAG is a primary regulator of insulin signaling [197], and that it antagonizes insulin action through various protein kinase C isoforms (e.g. PKC-θ) [198]. Indeed, DAG has been shown to accumulate in muscles obtained form insulin resistant rodents and humans [196,199]. Moreover, mice lacking the DAG-target PKC-θ are protected from insulin resistance caused by lipid infusion [198]. However, questions remain regarding whether DAG is the primary lipid metabolite accounting for insulin resistance in this experimental model, as well as whether it plays a quantitatively significant role in lipid-induced insulin resistance. First, phorbol esters which mimic DAG have often been shown to have no inhibitory effect in insulin action [200,201], Second, DAG produced after incubating cells with palmitate is insufficient to inhibit insulin signaling [67].

F6bii. Ceramides

Like DAG, ceramide has been shown to accumulate in some [202-205], but not all [197,199], experimental models of insulin resistance. Moreover, the sphingolipid has been shown to impair insulin signaling and glucose uptake through a number of different mechanisms, and to be a requisite intermediate linking the saturated fatty acid palmitate to the inhibition of insulin action. Thus, we favor a role for ceramide as one of possibly many lipid metabolites that impair glucose uptake and metabolism.

Inhibition of Insulin Signaling and Action by Ceramides- Ceramide acutely inhibits insulin-stimulated glucose uptake, GLUT4 translocation, and/or glycogen synthesis in cultured adipocytes and/or isolated skeletal muscle [131,206,207]. These effects appear to result from the sphingolipid's ability to block activation of either IRS-1 or Akt/PKB. Specifically, in 1996, two independent laboratories found that treating cultured cells with short-chain ceramide analogs or bacterial sphingomyelinases, which hydrolyze sphingomyelin to form choline and ceramide, blocked insulin-stimulated tyrosine phosphorylation of IRS-1 and its subsequent recruitment and activation of PI3-kinase [134,208]. A third group found that ceramide directly inhibited PI3-kinase isolated from serum-stimulated cells [209]. However, the effect of ceramide on IRS and/or PI3-kinase appears to be specific to certain cells or treatment conditions, as a number of different laboratories have shown that ceramide has no effect on PI3-kinase or the production of its lipid products [67,131,132,207,210]. In all cell types tested, however, ceramide has been shown to block activation of Akt/PKB [67,131-133,211-213]. Moreover, prolonged treatment of 3T3-L1 adipocytes with ceramide was additionally shown to decrease GLUT4 expression [214].

Role of Ceramides in FFA-Induced Insulin Resistance - To evaluate the role of ceramides in the insulin resistance associated with lipid oversupply, scientists have investigated the sphingolipid's role in FFA-induced insulin resistance using cultured myotubes. Schmitz-Pfeiffer et al. [215] first observed that treating C2C12's with saturated FFAs increased the intracellular pool of ceramide while simultaneously inhibiting activation of Akt/PKB, but not PI3-kinase, in C2C12 myotubes. In this cell type, short-chain ceramide analogs recapitulated this pattern of effects on insulin signal transduction, and the authors speculated that ceramide was the primary intermediate linking FFAs to the inhibition of insulin signaling. Using inhibitors of ceramide synthesis or overexpression strategies to prevent ceramide accumulation, we have demonstrated that blocking FFA-induced ceramide accumulation prevents their-inhibition of Akt/PKB, while blocking ceramide degradation exacerbates this FFA effect [67].

Molecular Mechanisms of Ceramide Action - The mechanisms by which sphingolipids, particularly ceramides, regulate cell function is controversial, as some researchers have argued that they function as traditional signaling molecules [216], while others have speculated that they elicit the majority of their effects by biophysically altering the plasma membrane [217]. Several ceramide targets have been considered as putative intermediates linking the sphingolipid to the inhibition of insulin signaling.

- *Protein Phosphatase 2A* – PP2A is one of the most highly expressed phosphatases, comprising 0.3 to 1% of cellular protein, and the enzyme is responsible for dephosphorylating a wide array of cellular phosphoproteins [218]. In particular, PP2A is the primary phosphatase responsible for dephosphorylating Akt/PKB in rat adipocytes [219], and inactivating PP2A in 3T3-L1 adipocytes augments insulin-stimulation of Akt/PKB activation, glucose uptake, and GLUT4 translocation [220]. Ceramide has been shown to activate both PP2A and PP1 *in vitro* [221]. Moreover, several groups have shown that the PP2A inhibitor okadaic acid can prevent various ceramide-mediated events [132,213,222,223], including its regulation of Akt/PKB [133]. As described previously, we also found that overexpressing the SV40 small T antigen, which displaces B-subunits within PP2A, also prevents ceramide effects on Akt/PKB [67,133].
- *Protein Kinase Cζ* - PDK1 phosphorylates a regulatory residue on PKC isoforms λ and ζ [224], which are serine/threonine kinases that also bind 3'-phosphoinositides, but do not contain recognizable PH-domains [225]. Experiments with constitutively active and dominant-negative forms of these enzymes support their involvement in insulin regulation of glucose uptake and GLUT4 translocation [226,227], but opposite findings are also reported [228]. In apparent contrast to PKCζ's role as a positive regulator of insulin-stimulated anabolic metabolism, reports identify the kinase as an intermediate linking ceramide to the inhibition of insulin action [229]. Specifically, ceramide has been shown to activate PKCζ in vitro [229], and inhibitors of the enzyme prevent its antagonism of Akt/PKB and glucose transport [211,230].
- *MLK3 and its targets JNK and IκKβ* - Mixed lineage kinase 3 is a member of the MAPKKK family that can activate JNK [231] and IκKβ [232], which are implicated

in insulin resistance. Ceramide has been shown to activate MLK3 [231], suggesting that it may serve as a primary regulator of lipid-induced insulin resistance.

F7. ER Stress

The endoplasmic reticulum (ER) is vulnerable to metabolic stresses, and this organelle may play a role in the etiology of insulin resistance [233-235]. Markers of ER stress are increased with obesity and are especially evident in obese mice that are fed a high-fat diet or are deficient in leptin [235]. The artificial induction of ER stress with the pharmacologic ER inhibitor tunicamycin has been shown to antagonize insulin signaling in cultured Fao hepatocytes, suggesting that ER stress may be sufficient to induce the insulin resistant state [235]. The precise mechanisms by which metabolic insults induce ER stress remain to be determined, but JNK has been identified as an intermediate linking tunicamycin to the antagonism of insulin signaling.

While ER stress may be sufficient to induce insulin resistance, recent studies suggest that it may not be required. Specifically, rats fed a high sucrose (HS) or high saturated fat (HSF) diet, but not a high polyunsaturated fat (HPF) one, developed ER stress [236]. When compared to controls, however, all three test groups displayed insulin resistance to the same extent. These data illustrate that ER stress is not requisite for the development of insulin resistance.

F8. Oxidative Stress and Reactive Oxygen Species

Reactive oxygen species (ROS) are oxygen-containing free radicals that are produced as a byproduct of mitochondrial fuel oxidation. Accumulation of these molecules causes oxidative stress and cellular damage by oxidizing lipids, proteins, and DNA within and outside of the mitochondria. Cells have the capacity to neutralize ROS with antioxidant enzymes such as superoxide dismutase and glutathione, and they have repair enzymes that can correct or replace ROS-damaged molecules. However, when the accumulation of cellular ROS exceeds the capacity for the cells to handle them then oxidative damage accumulates and mitochondrial function becomes impaired, resulting in loss of energy production [237-239].

Three models of insulin resistance; including glucocorticoid and TNFα treatment in adipocytes, and the db/db mouse model are all significantly protected from insulin resistance by a reduction of free radical stress [240]. Although the pathways by which glucocorticoids and TNFα cause insulin resistance are distinct, they do have the commonality of ceramide production. Ceramide is the possible missing link since it is capable of increasing mitochondrial ROS production. Nevertheless, cumulative mitochondrial and nuclear damage caused by ROS is typical with ageing, and may be one reason that ageing is also correlated with insulin resistance.

G. Perspective on Insulin Resistance and Treatment

Insulin resistance may have evolved as a protective mechanism that prevents glucose uptake and lipid production in non-adipose tissues, which, as evidenced from lipodystrophic models, can wreak havoc with organ function [241]. This comes at the price of elevated circulating glucose and insulin levels, but it provides a window of time to correct for obesity, poor diet, or inflammation. If left untreated, chronic insulin resistance has negative effects on metabolic and vascular properties, and places patients at risk for cardiovascular disease, diabetes, and certain forms of cancer.

At this time, the best treatment for insulin resistance and obesity is improved diet, reduced caloric intake, and exercise. These healthy lifestyle adjustments decrease body fat, combat inflammation, increase fat oxidation in lean tissues, lower muscle ceramide and DAG levels, promote skeletal muscle hypertrophy (which increases lipid and glucose utilization), and reduce blood glucose levels [242-245]. In fact, a single exercise session may increase insulin sensitivity for 16 hours or more [246-249]. Pharmaceuticals have been developed to mimic some of the effects of exercise (e.g. metformin, which activates AMPK to promote lipid oxidation), but none remain as wholly beneficial as a dedicated workout regimen with reduced caloric intake.

As described in this chapter, a wide variety of systems interact to control glucose homeostasis, and a number of different metabolic insults may contribute to insulin resistance. However, what is also clear is that we don't have a good appreciation for how these systems interact, and how changing one component alters the entire metabolic rheostat. Moreover, in any given individual, we don't understand which of these metabolic abnormalities play the largest quantitative role in the antagonism of insulin action. Researchers are currently addressing these more daunting questions, which will enable more precise treatment strategies for obesity-induced metabolic dysfunction.

H. Selected References

[1.] Bray, G. A. (2003) *Endocrinol. Metab. Clin. North. Am. 32(4)*, 787-804, viii

[2.] Cooney, K. A., and Gruber, S. B. (2005) *Jama 293(2)*, 235-236

[3.] Luzi, L., Giordano, M., Caloni, and Castellino, P. (2001) *Eur. J. Nutr. 40(3)*, 106-112

[4.] Dugani, C. B., and Klip, A. (2005) *EMBO Rep. 6(12)*, 1137-1142

[5.] Hausdorff, S. F., Fingar, D. C., Morioka, K., Garza, L. A., Whiteman, E. L., Summers, S. A., and Birnbaum, M. J. (1999) *J. Biol. Chem. 274(35)*, 24677-24684

[6.] Minokoshi, Y., Kahn, C. R., and Kahn, B. B. (2003) *J. Biol. Chem.* 278(36), 33609-33612

[7.] Ortmeyer, H. K. (1997*) J. Basic. Clin. Physiol. Pharmacol. 8(4)*, 223-235

[8.] Ortmeyer, H. K. (1997) *Obes. Res. 5(6)*, 613-621

[9.] Brady, M. J., Bourbonais, F. J., and Saltiel, A. R. (1998) *Journal of Biological Chemistry 273(23)*, 14063-14068

[10.] Roach, P. J. (2002) *Curr. Mol. Med. 2(2)*, 101-120

[11.] Asnaghi, L., Bruno, P., Priulla, M., and Nicolin, A. (2004) *Pharmacol. Res. 50(6)*, 545-549

[12.] Bullo, M., Garcia-Lorda, P., Peinado-Onsurbe, J., Hernandez, M., Del Castillo, D., Argiles, J. M., and Salas-Salvado, J. (2002) *Int. J. Obes. Relat. Metab. Disord. 26(5)*, 652-658

[13.] Romsos, D. R., and Leveille, G. A. (1974) *Proc. Soc. Exp. Biol. Med. 145(2)*, 591-594

[14.] Romsos, D. R., and Leveille, G. A. (1974) *Adv. Lipid. Res. 12(0)*, 97-146

[15.] Park, S. Y., Kim, H. J., Wang, S., Higashimori, T., Dong, J., Kim, Y. J., Cline, G., Li, H., Prentki, M., Shulman, G. I., Mitchell, G. A., and Kim, J. K. (2005) *Am. J. Physiol. Endocrinol. Metab.*

[16.] Belfrage, P., Fredrikson, G., Nilsson, N. O., and Stralfors, P. (1981) *Int. J. Obes. 5(6)*, 635-641

[17.] Smith, C. J., and Manganiello, V. C. (1989) *Mol. Pharmacol. 35(3)*, 381-386

[18.] Radziuk, J., and Pye, S. (2001) *Diabetes Metab. Res. Rev. 17(4)*, 250-272

[19.] Postic, C., Dentin, R., and Girard, J. (2004) *Diabetes Metab. 30(5)*, 398-408

[20.] Oberkofler, H., Klein, K., Felder, T. K., Krempler, F., and Patsch, W. (2006) *Endocrinology 147(2)*, 966-976

[21.] Oberkofler, H., Schraml, E., Krempler, F., and Patsch, W. (2004) *Biochem. J. 381(Pt 2)*, 357-363

[22.] Triggle, C. R., Ding, H., Anderson, T. J., and Pannirselvam, M. (2004) *Mol. Cell Biochem. 263(1-2)*, 21-27

[23.] Wilcox, C. S. (2005) *Am. J. Physiol. Regul. Integr. Comp. Physiol. 289(4)*, R913-935

[24.] Fulton, D., Gratton, J. P., McCabe, T. J., Fontana, J., Fujio, Y., Walsh, K., Franke, T. F., Papapetropoulos, A., and Sessa, W. C. (1999) *Nature 399(6736)*, 597-601

[25.] Hattori, S., Hattori, Y., and Kasai, K. (2005) *Metabolism 54(4)*, 482-487

[26.] Hattori, Y., Suzuki, M., Hattori, S., and Kasai, K. (2003) *Diabetologia 46(11)*, 1543-1549

[27.] Leighton, F., Miranda-Rottmann, S., and Urquiaga, I. (2005) *Cell Biochem. Funct,* epub ahead of print

[28.] Sanchez, M., Galisteo, M., Vera, R., Villar, I. C., Zarzuelo, A., Tamargo, J., Perez-Vizcaino, F., and Duarte, J. (2006) *J. Hypertens 24(1)*, 75-84

[29.] Toba, H., Nakagawa, Y., Miki, S., Shimizu, T., Yoshimura, A., Inoue, R., Asayama, J., Kobara, M., and Nakata, T. (2005) *Hypertens Res. 28(8)*, 689-700

[30.] Duplain, H., Burcelin, R., Sartori, C., Cook, S., Egli, M., Lepori, M., Vollenweider, P., Pedrazzini, T., Nicod, P., Thorens, B., and Scherrer, U. (2001) *Circulation 104(3)*, 342-345

[31.] Shankar, R. R., Wu, Y., Shen, H. Q., Zhu, J. S., and Baron, A. D. (2000) *Diabetes 49(5)*, 684-687

[32.] Siddle, K., Urso, B., Niesler, C. A., Cope, D. L., Molina, L., Surinya, K. H., and Soos, M. A. (2001) *Biochem. Soc. Trans. 29(Pt 4)*, 513-525

[33.] Liu, S. C., Wang, Q., Lienhard, G. E., and Keller, S. R. (1999) *J. Biol. Chem. 274(25)*, 18093-18099

[34.] Kido, Y., Burks, D. J., Withers, D., Bruning, J. C., Kahn, C. R., White, M. F., and Accili, D. (2000) *J. Clin. Invest. 105(2)*, 199-205

[35.] Fantin, V. R., Wang, Q., Lienhard, G. E., and Keller, S. R. (2000) *Am. J. Physiol. Endocrinol. Metab. 278(1)*, E127-133

[36.] Gual, P., Le Marchand-Brustel, Y., and Tanti, J. F. (2005) *Biochimie 87(1)*, 99-109

[37.] Alessi, D. R., James, S. R., Downes, C. P., Holmes, A. B., Gaffney, P. R., Reese, C. B., and Cohen, P. (1997) *Current Biology 7(4)*, 261-269

[38.] Sarbassov, D. D., Guertin, D. A., Ali, S. M., and Sabatini, D. M. (2005) *Science 307(5712)*, 1098-1101

[39.] Leslie, N. R., Biondi, R. M., and Alessi, D. R. (2001) *Chem. Rev. 101(8)*, 2365-2380

[40.] Brazil, D. P., and Hemmings, B. A. (2001) *Trends Biochem. Sci. 26(11)*, 657-664.

[41.] Jiang, Z. Y., Zhou, Q. L., Coleman, K. A., Chouinard, M., Boese, Q., and Czech, M. P. (2003) *Proc. Natl. Acad. Sci. U S A 100(13)*, 7569-7574.

[42.] Hill, M. M., Clark, S. F., Tucker, D. F., Birnbaum, M. J., James, D. E., and Macaulay, S. L. (1999) *Mol. Cell Biol. 19(11)*, 7771-7781

[43.] Zhou, Q. L., Park, J. G., Jiang, Z. Y., Holik, J. J., Mitra, P., Semiz, S., Guilherme, A., Powelka, A. M., Tang, X., Virbasius, J., and Czech, M. P. (2004) *Biochem. Soc. Trans. 32(Pt 5)*, 817-821

[44.] van Dam, E. M., Govers, R., and James, D. E. (2005) *Mol Endocrinol 19(4)*, 1067-1077

[45.] Kohn, A. D., Summers, S. A., Birnbaum, M. J., and Roth, R. A. (1996) *J. Biol. Chem. 271(49)*, 31372-31378

[46.] Egawa, K., Sharma, P. M., Nakashima, N., Huang, Y., Huver, E., Boss, G. R., and Olefsky, J. M. (1999) *J. Biol. Chem. 274(20)*, 14306-14314

[47.] Kane, S., Sano, H., Liu, S. C., Asara, J. M., Lane, W. S., Garner, C. C., and Lienhard, G. E. (2002) *J. Biol. Chem. 277(25)*, 22115-22118

[48.] Zeigerer, A., McBrayer, M. K., and McGraw, T. E. (2004) *Mol. Biol. Cell 15(10)*, 4406-4415

[49.] Bruss, M. D., Arias, E. B., Lienhard, G. E., and Cartee, G. D. (2005) *Diabetes 54(1)*, 41-50

[50.] Welsh, G. I., Hers, I., Berwick, D. C., Dell, G., Wherlock, M., Birkin, R., Leney, S., and Tavare, J. M. (2005) *Biochem. Soc. Trans. 33(Pt 2)*, 346-349

[51.] Khan, A. H., and Pessin, J. E. (2002) *Diabetologia 45(11)*, 1475-1483

[52.] Chiang, S. H., Hou, J. C., Hwang, J., Pessin, J. E., and Saltiel, A. R. (2002) *J. Biol. Chem. 277(15)*, 13067-13073

[53.] Watson, R. T., Shigematsu, S., Chiang, S. H., Mora, S., Kanzaki, M., Macara, I. G., Saltiel, A. R., and Pessin, J. E. (2001) *J. Cell Biol. 154(4)*, 829-840

[54.] Chiang, S. H., Baumann, C. A., Kanzaki, M., Thurmond, D. C., Watson, R. T., Neudauer, C. L., Macara, I. G., Pessin, J. E., and Saltiel, A. R. (2001) *Nature 410(6831)*, 944-948

[55.] Molero, J. C., Jensen, T. E., Withers, P. C., Couzens, M., Herzog, H., Thien, C. B., Langdon, W. Y., Walder, K., Murphy, M. A., Bowtell, D. D., James, D. E., and Cooney, G. J. (2004) *J. Clin. Invest. 114(9)*, 1326-1333

[56.] Mitra, P., Zheng, X., and Czech, M. P. (2004) *J. Biol. Chem. 279(36)*, 37431-37435

[57.] Chang, L., Chiang, S. H., and Saltiel, A. R. (2005) *Mol. Med.* 406:701-14.

[58.]   Dickson, L. M., and Rhodes, C. J. (2004) *Am. J. Physiol. Endocrinol. Metab. 287(2)*, E192-198

[59.]   Ascott-Evans, B. H. (2005) *Sadj. 60(3)*, 122, 127

[60.]   Issa, B. G., and Hanna, F. W. (2003) *Curr. Opin. Lipidol. 14(4)*, 405-407

[61.]   Grundy, S. M., Cleeman, J. I., Daniels, S. R., Donato, K. A., Eckel, R. H., Franklin, B. A., Gordon, D. J., Krauss, R. M., Savage, P. J., Smith, S. C., Jr., Spertus, J. A., and Costa, F. (2005) *Circulation 112(17)*, 2735-2752

[62.]   Ruderman, N. B., Schneider, S. H., and Berchtold, P. (1981) *Am. J. Clin. Nutr. 34(8)*, 1617-1621

[63.]   Curat, C. A., Miranville, A., Sengenes, C., Diehl, M., Tonus, C., Busse, R., and Bouloumie, A. (2004) *Diabetes 53(5)*, 1285-1292

[64.]   Guo, K. Y., Halo, P., Leibel, R. L., and Zhang, Y. (2004) *Am. J. Physiol. Regul. Integr. Comp. Physiol. 287(1)*, R112-119

[65.]   Winkler, G., Kiss, S., Keszthelyi, L., Sapi, Z., Ory, I., Salamon, F., Kovacs, M., Vargha, P., Szekeres, O., Speer, G., Karadi, I., Sikter, M., Kaszas, E., Dworak, O., Gero, G., and Cseh, K. (2003*) Eur. J. Endocrinol. 149(2)*, 129-135

[66.]   McGarry, J. D. (1995) *Curr. Biol. 5(12)*, 1342-1344.

[67.]   Chavez, J. A., Knotts, T. A., Wang, L. P., Li, G., Dobrowsky, R. T., Florant, G. L., and Summers, S. A. (2003) *J. Biol. Chem. 278(12)*, 10297-10303.

[68.]   Borst, S. E. (2004) *Endocrine 23(2-3)*, 177-182

[69.]   McGarry, J. D. (2002) *Diabetes 51(1)*, 7-18

[70.]   Tang, Y., Osawa, H., Onuma, H., Nishimiya, T., Ochi, M., Sugita, A., and Makino, H. (2001) *Diabetes Res. Clin. Pract. 54(3)*, 145-155

[71.]   Smith, S. R., Lovejoy, J. C., Greenway, F., Ryan, D., deJonge, L., de la Bretonne, J., Volafova, J., and Bray, G. A. (2001) *Metabolism 50(4)*, 425-435

[72.]   Klein, S. (2004) *J. Clin. Invest. 113(11)*, 1530-1532

[73.]   Freedland, E. S. (2004) *Nutr. Metab. (Lond) 1(1)*, 12

[74.]   Busetto, L. (2001) *Nutr. Metab. Cardiovasc. Dis. 11(3)*, 195-204

[75.]   Janssen, I., Katzmarzyk, P. T., Ross, R., Leon, A. S., Skinner, J. S., Rao, D. C., Wilmore, J. H., Rankinen, T., and Bouchard, C. (2004) *Obes. Res. 12(3)*, 525-537

[76.]   Goodpaster, B. H., Kelley, D. E., Wing, R. R., Meier, A., and Thaete, F. L. (1999) *Diabetes 48(4)*, 839-847

[77.]   Kamel, E. G., McNeill, G., and Van Wijk, M. C. (2000) *Int. J. Obes. Relat. Metab. Disord. 24(5)*, 607-613

[78.]   Unger, R. H. (2003) *Endocrinology 144(12)*, 5159-5165

[79.]   Nolan, D., and Mallal, S. (2001) *Aids 15(15)*, 2037-2041

[80.]   Vigouroux, C., Gharakhanian, S., Salhi, Y., Nguyen, T. H., Adda, N., Rozenbaum, W., and Capeau, J. (1999) *Diabetes Metab 25(5)*, 383-392

[81.]   Vigouroux, C., Gharakhanian, S., Salhi, Y., Nguyen, T. H., Chevenne, D., Capeau, J., and Rozenbaum, W. (1999) *Diabetes Metab. 25(3)*, 225-232

[82.]   Colombo, C., Cutson, J. J., Yamauchi, T., Vinson, C., Kadowaki, T., Gavrilova, O., and Reitman, M. L. (2002) *Diabetes 51(9)*, 2727-2733

[83.]   Poehlman, E. T., Toth, M. J., and Gardner, A. W. (1995) *Ann. Intern. Med. 123(9)*, 673-675

[84.] Carr, M. C. (2003) *J. Clin. Endocrinol. Metab. 88(6)*, 2404-2411

[85.] Weber, R. V., Buckley, M. C., Fried, S. K., and Kral, J. G. (2000) *Am. J. Physiol. Regul. Integr. Comp. Physiol. 279(3)*, R936-943

[86.] Barzilai, N., She, L., Liu, B. Q., Vuguin, P., Cohen, P., Wang, J., and Rossetti, L. (1999) *Diabetes 48(1)*, 94-98

[87.] D'Andrea, F., Grella, R., Rizzo, M. R., Grella, E., Grella, R., Nicoletti, G., Barbieri, M., and Paolisso, G. (2005) *Aesthetic Plast. Surg.* 29(6):472-8; discussion 479-80, 481

[88.] Arner, P. (2004) *N. Engl. J. Med. 351(13)*, 1354-1357; author reply 1354-1357

[89.] Busetto, L., Bassetto, F., and Nolli, M. L. (2004) *N. Engl. J. Med. 351(13)*, 1354-1357; author reply 1354-1357

[90.] Esposito, K., Giugliano, G., and Giugliano, D. (2004) *N. Engl. J. Med. 351(13)*, 1354-1357; author reply 1354-1357

[91.] Klein, S., Fontana, L., Young, V. L., Coggan, A. R., Kilo, C., Patterson, B. W., and Mohammed, B. S. (2004) *N. Engl. J. Med. 350(25)*, 2549-2557

[92.] Minocci, A., Savia, G., Lucantoni, R., Berselli, M. E., Tagliaferri, M., Calo, G., Petroni, M. L., de Medici, C., Viberti, G. C., and Liuzzi, A. (2000) *Int. J. Obes. Relat. Metab. Disord. 24(9)*, 1139-1144

[93.] Unger, R. H. (2003) *Trends Endocrinol. Metab. 14(9)*, 398-403

[94.] Frayn, K. N. (2000) *Br. J. Nutr. 83 Suppl 1*, S71-77

[95.] Nielsen, S., Guo, Z., Johnson, C. M., Hensrud, D. D., and Jensen, M. D. (2004) *J. Clin. Invest. 113(11)*, 1582-1588

[96.] Lundgren, M., Buren, J., Ruge, T., Myrnas, T., and Eriksson, J. W. (2004) *J. Clin. Endocrinol. Metab. 89(6)*, 2989-2997

[97.] Kahn, B. B. (1994) *J. Nutr. 124(8 Suppl)*, 1289S-1295S

[98.] Tozzo, E., Shepherd, P. R., Gnudi, L., and Kahn, B. B. (1995) *Am. J. Physiol. 268(5 Pt 1)*, E956-964

[99.] Qin Yang, T. E. G., Nimesh Mody, Frederic Preitner, Odile D. Peroni, Janice M. Zabolotny, Ko Kotani, Loredana Quadro and Barbara B. Kahn. (2005) *Nature 436*, 356-362

[100.] Bujalska, I. J., Kumar, S., and Stewart, P. M. (1997) *Lancet 349(9060)*, 1210-1213

[101.] Bjorntorp, P. (1995) *Metabolism 44(9 Suppl 3)*, 21-23

[102.] Masuzaki, H., Paterson, J., Shinyama, H., Morton, N. M., Mullins, J. J., Seckl, J. R., and Flier, J. S. (2001) *Science 294(5549)*, 2166-2170

[103.] Paterson, J. M., Morton, N. M., Fievet, C., Kenyon, C. J., Holmes, M. C., Staels, B., Seckl, J. R., and Mullins, J. J. (2004) *Proc. Natl. Acad. Sci. U S A 101(18)*, 7088-7093

[104.] Hermanowski-Vosatka, A., Balkovec, J. M., Cheng, K., Chen, H. Y., Hernandez, M., Koo, G. C., Le Grand, C. B., Li, Z., Metzger, J. M., Mundt, S. S., Noonan, H., Nunes, C. N., Olson, S. H., Pikounis, B., Ren, N., Robertson, N., Schaeffer, J. M., Shah, K., Springer, M. S., Strack, A. M., Strowski, M., Wu, K., Wu, T., Xiao, J., Zhang, B. B., Wright, S. D., and Thieringer, R. (2005) *J. Exp. Med. 202(4)*, 517-527

[105.] Kershaw, E. E., Morton, N. M., Dhillon, H., Ramage, L., Seckl, J. R., and Flier, J. S. (2005) *Diabetes 54(4)*, 1023-1031

[106.] Wellen, K. E., and Hotamisligil, G. S. (2005) *J. Clin. Invest. 115(5)*, 1111-1119

[107.] Cinti, S., Mitchell, G., Barbatelli, G., Murano, I., Ceresi, E., Faloia, E., Wang, S., Fortier, M., Greenberg, A. S., and Obin, M. S. (2005) *J. Lipid. Res. 46(11)*, 2347-2355

[108.] Tarkun, I., Cetinarslan, B., Turemen, E., Sahin, T., Canturk, Z., and Komsuoglu, B. (2005) *Eur. J. Endocrinol. 153(1)*, 115-121

[109.] Blum, C. A., Muller, B., Huber, P., Kraenzlin, M., Schindler, C., De Geyter, C., Keller, U., and Puder, J. J. (2005) *J. Clin. Endocrinol. Metab. 90(6)*, 3230-3235

[110.] Hirosumi, J., Tuncman, G., Chang, L., Gorgun, C. Z., Uysal, K. T., Maeda, K., Karin, M., and Hotamisligil, G. S. (2002) *Nature 420(6913)*, 333-336

[111.] Uysal, K. T., Wiesbrock, S. M., and Hotamisligil, G. S. (1998) *Endocrinology 139(12)*, 4832-4838

[112.] Ventre, J., Doebber, T., Wu, M., MacNaul, K., Stevens, K., Pasparakis, M., Kollias, G., and Moller, D. E. (1997) *Diabetes 46(9)*, 1526-1531

[113.] Yuan, M., Konstantopoulos, N., Lee, J., Hansen, L., Li, Z. W., Karin, M., and Shoelson, S. E. (2001*) Science 293(5535)*, 1673-1677

[114.] Montague, C. T., Prins, J. B., Sanders, L., Zhang, J., Sewter, C. P., Digby, J., Byrne, C. D., and O'Rahilly, S. (1998) *Diabetes 47(9)*, 1384-1391

[115.] Hotamisligil, G. S., Arner, P., Atkinson, R. L., and Spiegelman, B. M. (1997) *Diabetes 46(3)*, 451-455

[116.] Moller, D. E. (2000) *Trends Endocrinol. Metab. 11(6)*, 212-217

[117.] Peraldi, P., and Spiegelman, B. M. (1997) *Journ. Annu. Diabetol. Hotel Dieu*, 149-159

[118.] Hotamisligil, G. S. (1999) *J. Intern. Med. 245(6)*, 621-625

[119.] Hotamisligil, G. S., Peraldi, P., Budavari, A., Ellis, R., White, M. F., and Spiegelman, B. M. (1996) *Science 271(5249)*, 665-668

[120.] Lang, C. H., Dobrescu, C., and Bagby, G. J. (1992) *Endocrinology 130(1)*, 43-52

[121.] Plomgaard, P., Bouzakri, K., Krogh-Madsen, R., Mittendorfer, B., Zierath, J. R., and Pedersen, B. K. (2005) *Diabetes 54(10)*, 2939-2945

[122.] Hotamisligil, G. S., Shargill, N. S., and Spiegelman, B. M. (1993) *Science 259(5091)*, 87-91

[123.] Tsigos, C., Kyrou, I., Chala, E., Tsapogas, P., Stavridis, J. C., Raptis, S. A., and Katsilambros, N. (1999) *Metabolism 48(10)*, 1332-1335

[124.] Moon, Y. S., Kim, D. H., and Song, D. K. (2004) *Metabolism 53(7)*, 863-867

[125.] Hotamisligil, G. S. (1999) *Exp. Clin. Endocrinol. Diabetes. 107(2)*, 119-125

[126.] Uysal, K. T., Wiesbrock, S. M., Marino, W. M., and Hotamisligil, G. S. (1997) *Nature 389*, 610-614

[127.] Ofei, F., Hurel, S., Newkirk, J., Sopwith, M., and Taylor, R. (1996) *Diabetes 45(7)*, 881-885

[128.] Sumida, M., Sekiya, K., Okuda, H., Tanaka, Y., and Shiosaka, T. (1990) *J. Biochem. (Tokyo) 107(1)*, 1-2

[129.] Stephens, J. M., and Pekala, P. H. (1992) *J. Biol. Chem. 267(19)*, 13580-13584

[130.] Ueki, K., Kondo, T., and Kahn, C. R. (2004) *Mol. Cell Biol. 24(12)*, 5434-5446

[131.] Summers, S. A., Garza, L. A., Zhou, H., and Birnbaum, M. J. (1998) *Mol. Cell Biol. 18(9)*, 5457-5464

[132.] Teruel, T., Hernandez, R., and Lorenzo, M. (2001) *Diabetes 50(11)*, 2563-2571.

[133.] Stratford, S., Hoehn, K. L., Liu, F., and Summers, S. A. (2004) *J. Biol. Chem. 279(35)*, 36608-36615

[134.] Peraldi, P., Hotamisligil, G. S., Buurman, W. A., White, M. F., and Spiegelman, B. M. (1996) *Journal of Biological Chemistry 271(22)*, 13018-13022

[135.] Rotter, V., Nagaev, I., and Smith, U. (2003) *J. Biol. Chem. 278(46)*, 45777-45784

[136.] Fried, S. K., Bunkin, D. A., and Greenberg, A. S. (1998) *J. Clin. Endocrinol. Metab. 83(3)*, 847-850

[137.] Church, T. S., Willis, M. S., Priest, E. L., Lamonte, M. J., Earnest, C. P., Wilkinson, W. J., Wilson, D. A., and Giroir, B. P. (2005) *Int. J. Obes. (Lond) 29(6)*, 675-681

[138.] Weisberg, S. P., McCann, D., Desai, M., Rosenbaum, M., Leibel, R. L., and Ferrante, A. W., Jr. (2003) *J Clin Invest 112(12)*, 1796-1808

[139.] Fain, J. N., Madan, A. K., Hiler, M. L., Cheema, P., and Bahouth, S. W. (2004) *Endocrinology 145(5)*, 2273-2282

[140.] Senn, J. J., Klover, P. J., Nowak, I. A., Zimmers, T. A., Koniaris, L. G., Furlanetto, R. W., and Mooney, R. A. (2003) *J Biol Chem 278(16)*, 13740-13746

[141.] Wallenius, V., Wallenius, K., Ahren, B., Rudling, M., Carlsten, H., Dickson, S. L., Ohlsson, C., and Jansson, J. O. (2002) *Nat Med 8(1)*, 75-79

[142.] Faldt, J., Wernstedt, I., Fitzgerald, S. M., Wallenius, K., Bergstrom, G., and Jansson, J. O. (2004) *Endocrinology 145(6)*, 2680-2686

[143.] Appel, S. J., Harrell, J. S., and Davenport, M. L. (2005) *J. Am. Acad. Nurse. Pract. 17(12)*, 535-541

[144.] Skurk, T., and Hauner, H. (2004) *Int. J. Obes. Relat. Metab. Disord. 28(11)*, 1357-1364

[145.] Liang, X., Kanjanabuch, T., Mao, S. L., Hao, C. M., Tang, Y. W., Declerck, P. J., Hasty, A. H., Wasserman, D. H., Fogo, A. B., and Ma, L. J. (2006) *Am. J. Physiol. Endocrinol. Metab. 290(1)*, E103-113

[146.] Ma, L. J., Mao, S. L., Taylor, K. L., Kanjanabuch, T., Guan, Y., Zhang, Y., Brown, N. J., Swift, L. L., McGuinness, O. P., Wasserman, D. H., Vaughan, D. E., and Fogo, A. B. (2004) *Diabetes 53(2)*, 336-346

[147.] Steppan, C. M., Bailey, S. T., Bhat, S., Brown, E. J., Banerjee, R. R., Wright, C. M., Patel, H. R., Ahima, R. S., and Lazar, M. A. (2001) *Nature 409(6818)*, 307-312

[148.] Lee, J. H., Chan, J. L., Yiannakouris, N., Kontogianni, M., Estrada, E., Seip, R., Orlova, C., and Mantzoros, C. S. (2003) *J. Clin. Endocrinol. Metab. 88(10)*, 4848-4856

[149.] Smith, S. R., Bai, F., Charbonneau, C., Janderova, L., and Argyropoulos, G. (2003) *Diabetes 52(7)*, 1611-1618

[150.] Nagaev, I., and Smith, U. (2001) *Biochem Biophys Res Commun 285(2)*, 561-564

[151.] Fain, J. N., Cheema, P. S., Bahouth, S. W., and Lloyd Hiler, M. (2003) *Biochem. Biophys. Res. Commun 300(3)*, 674-678

[152.] Palanivel, R., Maida, A., Liu, Y., and Sweeney, G. (2005) *Diabetologia*, 1-8

[153.] Heilbronn, L. K., Rood, J., Janderova, L., Albu, J. B., Kelley, D. E., Ravussin, E., and Smith, S. R. (2004) *J. Clin. Endocrinol. Metab. 89(4)*, 1844-1848

[154.] Conneely, K. N., Silander, K., Scott, L. J., Mohlke, K. L., Lazaridis, K. N., Valle, T. T., Tuomilehto, J., Bergman, R. N., Watanabe, R. M., Buchanan, T. A., Collins, F. S., and Boehnke, M. (2004) *Diabetologia 47(10)*, 1782-1788

[155.] Sentinelli, F., Romeo, S., Arca, M., Filippi, E., Leonetti, F., Banchieri, M., Di Mario, U., and Baroni, M. G. (2002) *Diabetes 51(3)*, 860-862

[156.] Bo, S., Gambino, R., Pagani, A., Guidi, S., Gentile, L., Cassader, M., and Pagano, G. F. (2005) *Int. J. Obes. (Lond) 29(11)*, 1315-1320

[157.] Friedman, J. M. (2002*) Nutr. Rev. 60(10 Pt 2)*, S1-14; discussion S68-84, 85-17

[158.] Halaas, J. L., Gajiwala, K. S., Maffei, M., Cohen, S. L., Chait, B. T., Rabinowitz, D., Lallone, R. L., Burley, S. K., and Friedman, J. M. (1995) *Science 269(5223)*, 543-546

[159.] Farooqi, I. S., Matarese, G., Lord, G. M., Keogh, J. M., Lawrence, E., Agwu, C., Sanna, V., Jebb, S. A., Perna, F., Fontana, S., Lechler, R. I., DePaoli, A. M., and O'Rahilly, S. (2002) *J. Clin. Invest. 110(8)*, 1093-1103

[160.] Oral, E. A., Simha, V., Ruiz, E., Andewelt, A., Premkumar, A., Snell, P., Wagner, A. J., DePaoli, A. M., Reitman, M. L., Taylor, S. I., Gorden, P., and Garg, A. (2002) *N Engl. J. Med. 346(8)*, 570-578

[161.] Heymsfield, S. B., Greenberg, A. S., Fujioka, K., Dixon, R. M., Kushner, R., Hunt, T., Lubina, J. A., Patane, J., Self, B., Hunt, P., and McCamish, M. (1999) *Jama 282(16)*, 1568-1575

[162.] Muller-Wieland, D., and Kotzka, J. (2002) *Ann. N. Y. Acad. Sci. 967*, 19-27

[163.] Solinas, G., Summermatter, S., Mainieri, D., Gubler, M., Pirola, L., Wymann, M. P., Rusconi, S., Montani, J. P., Seydoux, J., and Dulloo, A. G. (2004) *FEBS Lett 577(3)*, 539-544

[164.] Yildiz, B. O., and Haznedaroglu, I. C. (2005) *Int. J. Biochem. Cell. Biol.* 38(5-6):820-30

[165.] Zhang, Y., Guo, K. Y., Diaz, P. A., Heo, M., and Leibel, R. L. (2002) *Am. J. Physiol. Regul. Integr. Comp. Physiol. 282(1)*, R226-234

[166.] Wang, M. Y., Orci, L., Ravazzola, M., and Unger, R. H. (2005) *Proc. Natl. Acad. Sci. U S A 102(50)*, 18011-18016

[167.] de Luca, C., Kowalski, T. J., Zhang, Y., Elmquist, J. K., Lee, C., Kilimann, M. W., Ludwig, T., Liu, S. M., and Chua, S. C. (2005) *J. Clin. Invest. 115(12)*, 3484-3493

[168.] Carpenter, L. R., Farruggella, T. J., Symes, A., Karow, M. L., Yancopoulos, G. D., and Stahl, N. (1998) *Proc. Natl. Acad. Sci. U S A 95(11)*, 6061-6066

[169.] Bjorbak, C., Lavery, H. J., Bates, S. H., Olson, R. K., Davis, S. M., Flier, J. S., and Myers, M. G., Jr. (2000) *J. Biol. Chem. 275(51)*, 40649-40657

[170.] Zabolotny, J. M., Bence-Hanulec, K. K., Stricker-Krongrad, A., Haj, F., Wang, Y., Minokoshi, Y., Kim, Y. B., Elmquist, J. K., Tartaglia, L. A., Kahn, B. B., and Neel, B. G. (2002) *Dev. Cell. 2(4)*, 489-495

[171.] Munzberg, H., Bjornholm, M., Bates, S. H., and Myers, M. G., Jr. (2005) *Cell. Mol. Life Sci. 62(6)*, 642-652

[172.] Yang, G., Ge, H., Boucher, A., Yu, X., and Li, C. (2004*) Mol. Endocrinol. 18(6)*, 1354-1362

[173.] Zastrow, O., Seidel, B., Kiess, W., Thiery, J., Keller, E., Bottner, A., and Kratzsch, J. (2003) *Int. J. Obes. Relat. Metab. Disord. 27(12)*, 1472-1478

[174.] Yamamoto, Y., Hirose, H., Saito, I., Nishikai, K., and Saruta, T. (2004) *J. Clin. Endocrinol. Metab. 89(1)*, 87-90

[175.] Bruun, J. M., Lihn, A. S., Verdich, C., Pedersen, S. B., Toubro, S., Astrup, A., and Richelsen, B. (2003) *Am. J. Physiol. Endocrinol. Metab. 285(3)*, E527-533

[176.] Maeda, N., Shimomura, I., Kishida, K., Nishizawa, H., Matsuda, M., Nagaretani, H., Furuyama, N., Kondo, H., Takahashi, M., Arita, Y., Komuro, R., Ouchi, N., Kihara, S., Tochino, Y., Okutomi, K., Horie, M., Takeda, S., Aoyama, T., Funahashi, T., and Matsuzawa, Y. (2002) *Nat. Med. 8(7)*, 731-737

[177.] Combs, T. P., Pajvani, U. B., Berg, A. H., Lin, Y., Jelicks, L. A., Laplante, M., Nawrocki, A. R., Rajala, M. W., Parlow, A. F., Cheeseboro, L., Ding, Y. Y., Russell, R. G., Lindemann, D., Hartley, A., Baker, G. R., Obici, S., Deshaies, Y., Ludgate, M., Rossetti, L., and Scherer, P. E. (2004) *Endocrinology 145(1)*, 367-383

[178.] Yamauchi, T., Kamon, J., Waki, H., Imai, Y., Shimozawa, N., Hioki, K., Uchida, S., Ito, Y., Takakuwa, K., Matsui, J., Takata, M., Eto, K., Terauchi, Y., Komeda, K., Tsunoda, M., Murakami, K., Ohnishi, Y., Naitoh, T., Yamamura, K., Ueyama, Y., Froguel, P., Kimura, S., Nagai, R., and Kadowaki, T. (2003) *J. Biol. Chem. 278(4)*, 2461-2468

[179.] Pajvani, U. B., Du, X., Combs, T. P., Berg, A. H., Rajala, M. W., Schulthess, T., Engel, J., Brownlee, M., and Scherer, P. E. (2003) *J. Biol. Chem. 278(11)*, 9073-9085

[180.] Fisher, F. F., Trujillo, M. E., Hanif, W., Barnett, A. H., McTernan, P. G., Scherer, P. E., and Kumar, S. (2005) *Diabetologia 48(6)*, 1084-1087

[181.] Dessein, P. H., Joffe, B. I., and Stanwix, A. E. (2003) *J. Rheumatol. 30(7)*, 1403-1405

[182.] Koike, K. (2006) *Intervirology 49(1-2)*, 51-57

[183.] Kim, H. J., Kim, H. J., Lee, K. E., Kim, D. J., Kim, S. K., Ahn, C. W., Lim, S. K., Kim, K. R., Lee, H. C., Huh, K. B., and Cha, B. S. (2004) *Arch. Intern. Med. 164(19)*, 2169-2175

[184.] McCullough, A. J. (2002) *J. Clin. Gastroenterol 34(3)*, 255-262

[185.] Donati, G., Stagni, B., Piscaglia, F., Venturoli, N., Morselli-Labate, A. M., Rasciti, L., and Bolondi, L. (2004) *Gut 53(7)*, 1020-1023

[186.] Mynarcik, D. C., Combs, T., McNurlan, M. A., Scherer, P. E., Komaroff, E., and Gelato, M. C. (2002) *J. Acquir. Immune. Defic. Syndr. 31(5)*, 514-520

[187.] Vincent-Desplanques, D., Faivre-Defrance, F., Wemeau, J. L., and Vantyghem, M. C. (2005) *Rev. Med Interne. 26(11)*, 866-873

[188.] Chen, N., Liu, L., Zhang, Y., Ginsberg, H. N., and Yu, Y. H. (2005) *Diabetes 54(12)*, 3379-3386

[189.] Krssak, M., Falk Petersen, K., Dresner, A., DiPietro, L., Vogel, S. M., Rothman, D. L., Roden, M., and Shulman, G. I. (1999) *Diabetologia 42(1)*, 113-116.

[190.] Matthaei, S., Stumvoll, M., Kellerer, M., and Haring, H. U. (2000) *Endocr. Rev. 21(6)*, 585-618

[191.] Dresner, A., Laurent, D., Marcucci, M., Griffin, M. E., Dufour, S., Cline, G. W., Slezak, L. A., Andersen, D. K., Hundal, R. S., Rothman, D. L., Petersen, K. F., and Shulman, G. I. (1999) *J. Clin. Invest. 103(2),* 253-259

[192.] Kim, J. K., Fillmore, J. J., Chen, Y., Yu, C., Moore, I. K., Pypaert, M., Lutz, E. P., Kako, Y., Velez-Carrasco, W., Goldberg, I. J., Breslow, J. L., and Shulman, G. I. (2001) *Proc. Natl. Acad. Sci U S A 98(13)*, 7522-7527.

[193.] Ferreira, L. D., Pulawa, L. K., Jensen, D. R., and Eckel, R. H. (2001) *Diabetes 50(5)*, 1064-1068.

[194.] Randle, P. J., Garland, P. B., Hales, L. N., Newsholme, E. A. (1963) *Lancet i,* 785-789

[195.] Boden, G., She, P., Mozzoli, M., Cheung, P., Gumireddy, K., Reddy, P., Xiang, X., Luo, Z., and Ruderman, N. (2005) *Diabetes 54(12)*, 3458-3465

[196.] Montell, E., Turini, M., Marotta, M., Roberts, M., Noe, V., Ciudad, C. J., Mace, K., and Gomez-Foix, A. M. (2001) *Am. J. Physiol. Endocrinol. Metab. 280(2)*, E229-237.

[197.] Yu, C., Chen, Y., Cline, G. W., Zhang, D., Zong, H., Wang, Y., Bergeron, R., Kim, J. K., Cushman, S. W., Cooney, G. J., Atcheson, B., White, M. F., Kraegen, E. W., and Shulman, G. I. (2002) *J. Biol. Chem. 277(52)*, 50230-50236

[198.] Kim, J. K., Fillmore, J. J., Sunshine, M. J., Albrecht, B., Higashimori, T., Kim, D. W., Liu, Z. X., Soos, T. J., Cline, G. W., O'Brien, W. R., Littman, D. R., and Shulman, G. I. (2004) *J. Clin. Invest. 114(6)*, 823-827

[199.] Itani, S. I., Ruderman, N. B., Schmieder, F., and Boden, G. (2002) *Diabetes 51(7)*, 2005-2011

[200.] Sowell, M. O., Treutelaar, M. K., Burant, C. F., and Buse, M. G. (1988) *Diabetes 37(5)*, 499-506

[201.] Witters, L. A., Vater, C. A., and Lienhard, G. E. (1985) *Nature 315(6022)*, 777-778

[202.] Adams, J. M., 2nd, Pratipanawatr, T., Berria, R., Wang, E., DeFronzo, R. A., Sullards, M. C., and Mandarino, L. J. (2004) *Diabetes 53(1)*, 25-31

[203.] Gorska, M., Dobrzyn, A., Zendzian-Piotrowska, M., and Gorski, J. (2004) *Horm. Metab. Res. 36(1)*, 14-21

[204.] Straczkowski, M., Kowalska, I., Nikolajuk, A., Dzienis-Straczkowska, S., Kinalska, I., Baranowski, M., Zendzian-Piotrowska, M., Brzezinska, Z., and Gorski, J. (2004) *Diabetes 53(5)*, 1215-1221

[205.] Turinsky, J., O'Sullivan, D. M., and Bayly, B. P. (1990) *Journal of Biological Chemistry 265(28)*, 16880-16885

[206.] Hajduch, E., Alessi, D. R., Hemmings, B. A., and Hundal, H. S. (1998) *Diabetes 47(7)*, 1006-1013.

[207.] Wang, C.-N., O'Brien, L., and Brindley, D. N. (1998) *Diabetes 47*, 24-31

[208.] Kanety, H., Hemi, R., Papa, M. Z., and Karasik, A. (1996) *Journal of Biological Chemistry 271(17)*, 9895-9897

[209.] Zundel, W., and Giaccia, A. (1998) *Genes. Dev. 12(13)*, 1941-1946

[210.] Hajduch, E., Balendran, A., Batty, I. H., Litherland, G. J., Blair, A. S., Downes, C. P., and Hundal, H. S. (2001) *Diabetologia 44(2)*, 173-183.

[211.] Powell, D. J., Hajduch, E., Kular, G., and Hundal, H. S. (2003) *Mol. Cell. Biol. 23(21)*, 7794-7808

[212.] Stratford, S., DeWald, D. B., and Summers, S. A. (2001) *Biochem. J. 354(Pt 2)*, 359-368.

[213.] Zinda, M. J., Vlahos, C. J., and Lai, M. T. (2001) *Biochem. Biophys. Res. Commun 280(4)*, 1107-1115.

[214.] Long, S. D., and Pekala, P. H. (1996) *Biochemical Journal 319*, 179-184

[215.] Schmitz-Peiffer, C., Craig, D. L., and Bidn, T. J. (1999) *Journal of Biological Chemistry 274(34)*, 24202-24210

[216.] Hannun, Y. A., and Obeid, L. M. (2002) *J. Biol. Chem .277(29)*, 25847-25850

[217.] van Blitterswijk, W. J., van der Luit, A. H., Veldman, R. J., Verheij, M., and Borst, J. (2003) *Biochem J 369(Pt 2)*, 199-211

[218.] Virshup, D. M. (2000) *Curr Opin Cell Biol 12(2)*, 180-185

[219.] Resjo, S., Goransson, O., Harndahl, L., Zolnierowicz, S., Manganiello, V., and Degerman, E. (2002) *Cell Signal 14(3)*, 231-238.

[220.] Ugi, S., Imamura, T., Maegawa, H., Egawa, K., Yoshizaki, T., Shi, K., Obata, T., Ebina, Y., Kashiwagi, A., and Olefsky, J. M. (2004) *Mol. Cell Biol. 24(19)*, 8778-8789

[221.] Chalfant, C. E., Kishikawa, K., Mumby, M. C., Kamibayashi, C., Bielawska, A., and Hannun, Y. A. (1999) *J. Biol. Chem. 274(29)*, 20313-20317

[222.] Kowluru, A., and Metz, S. A. (1997) *FEBS Letters 418*, 179-182

[223.] Salinas, M., Lopez-Valdaliso, R., Martin, D., Alvarez, A., and Cuadrado, A. (2000) *Mol. Cell Neurosci. 15(2)*, 156-169

[224.] Chou, M. M., Hou, W., Johnson, J., Graham, L. K., Lee, M. H., Chen, C. S., Newton, A. C., Schaffhausen, B. S., and Toker, A. (1998) *Curr. Biol. 8(19)*, 1069-1077

[225.] Akimoto, K., Takahashi, R., Moriya, S., Nishioka, N., Takayanagi, J., Kimura, K., Fukui, Y., Osada, S., Mizuno, K., Hirai, S., Kazlauskas, A., and Ohno, S. (1996) *Embo J. 15(4)*, 788-798

[226.] Kotani, K., Ogawa, W., Matsumoto, M., Kitamura, T., Sakaue, H., Hino, Y., Miyake, K., Sano, W., Akimoto, K., Ohno, S., and Kasuga, M. (1998) *Mol. Cell Biol. 18(12)*, 6971-6982

[227.] Standaert, M. L., Galloway, L., Karnam, P., Bandyopadhyay, G., Moscat, J., and Farese, R. V. (1997) *Journal of Biological Chemistry 272(48)*, 30075-30082

[228.] Tsuru, M., Katagiri, H., Asano, T., Yamada, T., Ohno, S., Ogihara, T., and Oka, Y. (2002) *Am. J. Physiol. Endocrinol. Metab. 283(2)*, E338-345

[229.] Muller, G., Ayoub, M., Storz, P., Rennecke, J., Fabbro, D., and Pfizenmaier, K. (1995) *Embo J. 14(9)*, 1961-1969

[230.] Powell, D. J., Turban, S., Gray, A., Hajduch, E., and Hundal, H. S. (2004) *Biochem. J 382(Pt 2)*, 619-629

[231.] Sathyanarayana, P., Barthwal, M. K., Kundu, C. N., Lane, M. E., Bergmann, A., Tzivion, G., and Rana, A. (2002) *Mol. Cell 10(6)*, 1527-1533.

[232.] Hehner, S. P., Hofmann, T. G., Ushmorov, A., Dienz, O., Wing-Lan Leung, I., Lassam, N., Scheidereit, C., Droge, W., and Schmitz, M. L. (2000) *Mol. Cell Biol 20(7)*, 2556-2568.

[233.] Hotamisligil, G. S. (2005) *Diabetes 54 Suppl. 2*, S73-78

[234.] Kharroubi, I., Ladriere, L., Cardozo, A. K., Dogusan, Z., Cnop, M., and Eizirik, D. L. (2004) *Endocrinology 145(11)*, 5087-5096

[235.] Ozcan, U., Cao, Q., Yilmaz, E., Lee, A. H., Iwakoshi, N. N., Ozdelen, E., Tuncman, G., Gorgun, C., Glimcher, L. H., and Hotamisligil, G. S. (2004) *Science 306(5695)*, 457-461

[236.] Wang, D., Wei, Y., and Pagliassotti, M. J. (2005) *Endocrinology* epub, ahead of print

[237.] de Grey, A. D. (2005) *Rejuvenation Res.* 8(1), 13-17

[238.] Miwa, S., and Brand, M. D. (2003) *Biochem. Soc. Trans.* 31(Pt 6), 1300-1301

[239.] Wei, Y. H., and Lee, H. C. (2002) *Exp. Biol. Med. (Maywood)* 227(9), 671-682

[240.] Houstis, N., Rosen, E. D., and Lander, E. S. (2006) *Nature* 440(7086), 944-948

[241.] Oral, E. A. (2003) *Rev. Endocr. Metab. Disord. 4(1)*, 61-77

[242.] Fujii, N., Aschenbach, W. G., Musi, N., Hirshman, M. F., and Goodyear, L. J. (2004) *Proc. Nutr. Soc. 63(2)*, 205-210

[243.] Goodpaster, B. H., and Kelley, D. E. (2002) *Curr. Diab. Rep. 2(3)*, 216-222

[244.] Helge, J. W., Dobrzyn, A., Saltin, B., and Gorski, J. (2004) *Exp. Physiol. 89(1)*, 119-127

[245.] Dobrzyn, A., Knapp, M., and Gorski, J. (2004) *Acta. Physiol. Scand. 181(3)*, 313-319

[246.] Devlin, J. T., Hirshman, M., Horton, E. D., and Horton, E. S. (1987) *Diabetes 36(4)*, 434-439

[247.] Baynard, T., Franklin, R. M., Goulopoulou, S., Carhart, R., Jr., and Kanaley, J. A. (2005) *Metabolism 54(8)*, 989-994

[248.] Kirwan, J. P., and del Aguila, L. F. (2003) *Biochem Soc Trans 31(Pt 6)*, 1281-1285

[249.] Henriksen, E. J. (2002) *J .Appl. Physiol. 93(2)*, 788-796

In: Progress in Metabolic Syndrome Research
Editor: George T. Ulrig, pp. 75-87

ISBN 1-60021-179-8
© 2006 Nova Science Publishers, Inc.

Chapter III

The Prevention of Type 2 Diabetes Mellitus

Rosane Ness-Abramof[1,] and Caroline M. Apovian[2]*
[1]Endocrine Unit, Sapir Medical Center, Tel Aviv University, Israel;
[2]Division of Endocrinology, Diabetes, Nutrition and Metabolism, Boston Medical Center,
Boston University, Boston, MA, USA.

Abstract

Type 2 diabetes (type 2 DM) is strongly associated with obesity. The obesity epidemic
has been accompanied during the last decade by a 25% increase in the prevalence of type
2 DM.

Diabetes confers an increased risk of cardiovascular disease, kidney disease and
microvascular complications including nephropathy, retinopathy and neuropathy.
Glycemic and blood pressure control were both shown to decrease microvascular and
macrovascular risk in patients with but it was not until recently that it was shown that
can be prevented, or at least delayed by lifestyle changes and pharmacologic therapy.

Lifestyle changes, including weight reduction, an increase in fiber consumption among
other nutritional changes, and an increase in physical activity, was shown to be highly
effective in preventing type 2 DM in high risk patients with impaired glucose tolerance.
In the Diabetes Prevention Program Study, patients randomized to lifestyle changes had a
58% reduced risk for developing diabetes, compared to the control group, while patients
treated with metformin had a 31% risk reduction. Pharmacotherapy, specifically
metformin, was also shown to be effective in the prevention of type 2 DM, although less
so than lifestyle changes. Patients treated with orlistat, a lipase inhibitor, and lifestyle
changes had a 37% risk reduction for developing diabetes, while patients treated with
acarbose (an α-glusidase inhibitor), had a 25% risk reduction.

---

* Correspondence concerning this article should be addressed to Rosane Abramof Ness, Endocrine Unit Sapir
Medical Center Tchernikovsky 53, Kfar Saba-Israel 44262. Fax: 972-9-7471328; Email: rosane-
abramof.ness@clalit.org.il.

The diabetes epidemic poses a worldwide health challenge due to its severe health consequences. Presently, several drugs has been shown to effective in preventing type 2 DM and many others are now being evaluated for this role. Lifestyle changes have been shown to be the most effective diabetes prevention strategy, particularly in patients with IGT, and should be widely implemented as primary therapy.

Introduction

The prevalence of type 2 diabetes is increasing in epidemic proportions in the U.S. and worldwide [1-3]. The diabetes epidemic is best explained by the increasing prevalence of obesity. The term "diabesity" emphasizes the close relationship between the two diseases [4-6].

Diabetes is one of the most costly chronic diseases, with its complications resulting in substantial morbidity and mortality. Microvascular complications in patients with diabetes include retinopathy, nephropathy and neuropathy which are the leading cause of blindness, end stage renal disease and non traumatic amputations in the western world [7,8]. Patients with type 2 DM have a higher prevalence of hypertension and lipid abnormalities and are at higher risk for coronary heart disease, stroke and peripheral vascular disease [9]. In the United Kingdom Prospective Diabetes Study (UKPDS), 50% of newly diagnosed patients with type 2 DM had already evidence of microvascular or macrovascular disease [10].

There is solid evidence showing that good glycemic control in patients with diabetes prevents or delays the progression of diabetic microvascular complications [11,12]. In the UKPDS trial, overweight patients treated with metformin alone, had a 38% reduction in the incidence of cardiovascular disease, primarily as myocardial infarction, making metformin the only oral hypoglycemic drug proven to reduce cardiovascular risk in patients with type 2 DM [13].

Table 1. Criteria for the diagnosis of impaired fasting glucose (IFG)

Normal fasting glucose	FPG< 100 mg/dl (5.6 mmol/l)
Impaired fasting glucose	FPG 100-125 mg/dl (5.6-6.9 mmol/l)

Pre-diabetes is a term that describes patients that have blood glucose levels above normal but have not reached the present diagnostic glucose threshold for the diagnosis of diabetes. Patients with pre-diabetes may have impaired fasting glucose (IFG) or impaired glucose tolerance (IGT) [14]. Impaired fasting glucose is defined as a fasting blood glucose between 100-125 mg/dl (before 2003, IFG was defined as a fasting blood glucose between 110-125 mg/dl)(Table 1). IGT is diagnosed if blood glucose levels after an oral glucose tolerance test (OGTT) are between140-199 mg/dl (table 2). Although both groups manifest impaired glucose homeostasis, the two conditions are not interchangeable and the risk for developing type 2 DM seems to be higher in patients with IGT [15]. The cumulative risk for developing type 2 DM over 5-6 years can be as high as 38-65% in patients that have both IFG and IGT [16]. The cardiovascular morbidity and risk of death in IGT and IFT are increased substantially compared to normoglycemic subjects [17-19]. The cluster of cardiovascular risk factors are more prevalent in this group and in fact, impaired glucose homeostasis is one of the criteria for the diagnosis of the metabolic syndrome (table 3)[20]. The metabolic syndrome is a cluster of metabolic risk factors that confer a higher risk for developing diabetes and atherosclerotic cardiovascular disease (ASCVD). It is estimated that 27% of the adult US population have the metabolic syndrome [21].

Table 2. Criteria for the diagnosis of impaired glucose tolerance (IGT) in patients after an oral glucose tolerance

Normal glucose tolerance	2 hour postload glucose < 140 mg/dl (7.8 nmol/l)
Impaired glucose tolerance	2 hour postload glucose 140-199 mg/dl (7.8-11.1 mmol/l)

Table 3. Criteria for Clinical Diagnosis of the Metabolic Syndrome (any 3 of 5 constitute diagnosis of the metabolic syndrome)

Measure	Categorical Cutpoints
Elevated Waist Circumference	$\geq$ 102 cm ($\geq$ 40 inches) in men $\geq$ 88 cm ($\geq$ 35 inches) in women
Elevated triglycerides	$\geq$ 150 mg/dl (1.7 mmol/L) or on drug treatment for elevated triglycerides
Reduced HDL-C	< 40 mg/dl (1.03 mmol/L) in men < 50 mg/dl (1.3 mmol/L) in women Or on drug treatment for reduced HDL-C
Elevated blood pressure	$\geq$ 130 mm Hg systolic blood pressure or $\geq$ 85 mm Hg diastolic blood pressure or on antihypertensive drug treatment in a patient with a history of hypertension
Elevated fasting glucose	$\geq$ 100 mg/dl or On drug treatment for elevated glucose

Reprinted with permission ref [20].

The alarming increase in the prevalence of diabetes and its serious health consequences, led researches to investigate whether type 2 diabetes could be prevented. During the last decade, well designed, prospective, randomized trials were conducted with the goal of prevention of type 2 DM. Studies included the investigation of lifestyle changes and drug therapy in high risk individuals, with both strategies showing positive results with a 25-58% relative risk reduction [22]. Lifestyle changes were more effective than medical therapy for diabetes prevention, but presently new drugs are being evaluated in clinical trials.

Prevention of Type 2 DM Through Lifestyle Changes

The Da Qing Impaired glucose tolerance and Diabetes study was one of the first randomized-controlled trials (RCTs) to evaluate the effect of lifestyle change in the prevention of diabetes. In this study, a total of 557 patients with IGT were randomized to one of 3 intervention groupswhich included diet-only, exercise-only or diet and exercise plus a control group. The control group was given general information concerning diet and how to increase leisure time physical activity. The exercise intervention group was instructed to increase the quantity of exercise daily equivalent to 20-40 minutes of brisk walking (patients < 50 years of age were encouraged to exercise more). The dietary intervention group was given dietary instructions and set for a reduction of caloric intake (individualized according to BMI). The development of diabetes was confirmed if the fasting glucose was 140 mg/dl or higher (the glucose threshold for the diagnosis of diabetes at the time of the study) or if the 2-hour postprandial glucose was 200 mg/dl or higher. Patients were followed for 6 years. The cumulative incidence of diabetes in 530 patients that completed the study was 67.7% in the control group, 43.8% in the diet group, 41.1% in the exercise group and 46% in the combined exercise and diet group. Each treatment group was superior to the control group, although there was no statistical difference between the different treatment modalities [22].

The Finnish Diabetes Prevention Study is a RCT which included 522 middle aged men and women (40-65 years) with impaired glucose tolerance and a mean BMI of 31 kg/m^2. The intervention group received individual counseling to reduce weight by at least 5%, to lower total fat intake to less than 30% of total calories, to increase fiber intake to 15 gr/1000 kcal or greater and to exercise at least 30 minutes per day. An OGTT was performed annually. Subjects were followed for a mean of 3.2 years. The cumulative incidence of diabetes after 4 years was 11% in the intervention group and 23% in the control group, with a relative risk reduction of 58% in patients randomized to lifestyle changes [23].

The largest trial evaluating the effectiveness of lifestyle changes in the prevention of diabetes was the Diabetes Prevention Study. A total of 3234 patients of multiple ethnicities with IGT were randomly assigned to placebo, metformin (850 mg twice daily) or a lifestyle modification program with a goal of at least a 7% weight loss and at least 150 minutes of physical activity per week. Patients were followed for a mean of 2.8 years. The incidence of diabetes was 11.0, 7.8, and 4.8 cases per 100 person years in the placebo, metformin, and lifestyle group respectively. The lifestyle intervention group had a 58% lower incidence for progressing to diabetes compared with placebo group (figure 1)[24]. Recently, Orchard et al published the prevalence of the metabolic syndrome (according to ATP III guidelines) in the DPP population. The prevalence of the metabolic syndrome was 55%, 54% and 51% in the placebo, metformin and intensive lifestyle modification group (ILT), respectively. The prevalence of the metabolic syndrome increased in patients assigned to placebo (61%) while patients assigned to ILT had a reduction of 41% compared to the placebo group, and patients treated with metformin had a 29% reduction in the prevalence of the metabolic syndrome compared to placebo treated patients. Lifestyle intervention reduced the prevalence of all components of the metabolic syndrome, except for HDL reduction, while metformin reduced only the prevalence of elevated waist circumference and fasting blood glucose. It is not clear what the individual contribution of weight loss or increased physical activity is to the reduced prevalence of the metabolic syndrome in the DPP study. Nevertheless, the study shows that ILT is effective in reducing the prevalence of the metabolic syndrome in addition to the beneficial effect of diabetes prevention [25].

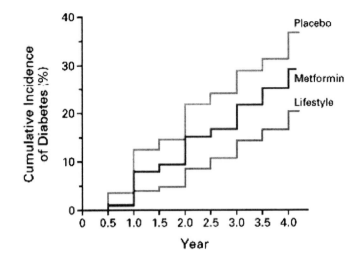

Figure 1. Cumulative Incidence of Diabetes According to Study Group. Reprinted with permission ref [24].

Pharmacological Therapy for the Prevention of Type 2 DM

Pharmacological therapy is an important therapeutic modality in the prevention of type 2 DM. Although lifestyle changes are highly effective in postponing or preventing type 2 DM it is doubtful if trial interventions can be replicated in real life and furthermore, permanent long term adherence to lifestyle changes are difficult to attain even in clinical trials.

Drug therapy to prevent type 2 DM has been investigated in randomized RCTs and in cohort studies. Most studies evaluated the effect of different oral hypoglycemics, antiobesity agents, antihypertensive agents, statins and fibrates for the prevention of type 2 DM [26].

Oral Hypoglycemic Agents for the Prevention of Type 2 DM

In the Diabetes Prevention Program (DPP), 2,155 individuals with IGT were randomized to metformin (850mg twice daily) or placebo (a third group as previously described, was randomized to intensive lifestyle changes) and were followed for a mean of 2.8 years [24]. In the placebo group, 7.8% of patients developed type 2 DM each year, while patients treated with metfomin had a 4.8% incidence of type 2 DM. Patients treated with metformin had a 31% risk reduction compared to placebo treated patients. In order to evaluate whether metformin prevented type 2 DM or merely unmasked it by early therapy, 79% of eligible patients had an oral glucose tolerance test (OGTT) after a 1-2 week washout period. The incidence of diabetes in the placebo group increased from 33.4% to 36.7% while in the metformin group there was a greater increase from 25.2 to 30.6% [27]. Even after a washout period, metformin still significantly decreased the relative risk for developing type 2 DM by 25%.

Acarbose, a α-glucosidase inhibitor, was studied in the Study to Prevent Noninsulin-Dependent Diabetes Mellitus (STOP-NIDDM) trial. Inclusion criteria included IGT and a fasting plasma glucose of 5.6-7.7 mmol/L (100-138 mg/dl) in order to increase the risk for diabetes progression. Patients were instructed on making lifestyle changes and randomized to receive acarbose 100 mg (714 subjects) or placebo (715 subjects) three times daily. The primary endpoint of the study was development of type 2 DM, evaluated by a yearly OGTT.

Patients were followed for a mean of 3.3 years. Thirty percent of patients treated with acarbose discontinued drug therapy due to side effects, which were mostly gastrointestinal. Patients whom did not develop diabetes were followed for an additional 3 months on placebo (single blind) and an OGTT was done at the end of this period. At the end of the study there was a 25% reduction in the risk for developing type 2 DM in patients treated with acarbose. Sixty percent of eligible patients had an OGTT after a 3 month washout period, with 15% of acarbose treated patients developing type 2 DM compared to 10.5% of patients on placebo. According to these results, acarbose therapy must be continued in order to exert its beneficial effect in diabetes prevention. It is possible that part of diabetes prevention during acarbose therapy is actually due to early treatment of type 2 DM. During the study period, acarbose increased reversion of IGT to normal glucose tolerance and in a secondary analysis, acarbose therapy reduced cardiovascular events from 4.7 to 2.1% [28,29].

The thiazolidinediones (TZDs) improve insulin action in muscle, adipose, and hepatic tissue by acting as agonists of the nuclear receptor peroxisome proliferator-activated recetor-γ (PPPAR-γ). Their effect is mediated by upregulation and downregulation of various genes resulting in improvement of lipid and glucose metabolism, vascular function and inflammatory response. By targeting insulin resistance, these drugs improve glucose control and there is also some evidence showing improvement in β-cell secretory function [30,31].

The Troglitazone in Prevention of Diabetes (TRIPOD) study [32] evaluated troglitazone therapy in prevention of diabetes. In this study, Hispanic women with a history of gestational diabetes were randomized to receive troglitazone, (a TZD), or placebo. After a median follow up of 30 months, the incidence of type 2 DM was 12.3% in placebo treated women and 5.4% in troglitazone treated patients, meaning a 56% reduction in progression to diabetes. This study was prematurely discontinued due to the withdrawal of troglitazone from the market due to severe hepatic toxicity. It is important to mention that after a washout period greater than 8 months, women treated with troglitazone still had a lower incidence of diabetes compared to placebo treated patients. This long-term effect of troglitazone in diabetes prevention favored a true preventive effect rather than early treatment of glucose intolerance. Unfortunately, the long-term effect of troglitazone on diabetes prevention was not replicated in the DPP trial. The DPP trial had a troglitazone arm that was prematurely discontinued in 1998 due to liver toxicity. During a mean follow up of 0.9 year, patients treated with troglitazone had a diabetes incidence of 3 cases/100 person-years, compared with 12, 6.7, and 5.1 cases/100 person years in the placebo, metformin and ILS participants, translating to a

75% risk reduction in developing diabetes in patients treated with troglitazone compared to placebo treatment. Patients were followed for 3 years after troglitazone withdrawal, during which the incidence of diabetes in this group was similar to the incidence in the placebo treated group. Therefore, according to this study, there is no evidence of a persistent protective effect of troglitazone in the prevention of diabetes [33].

Durbin [34] conducted a cohort study in which 101 patients with IGT or insulin resistance (IR) were treated with troglitazone for a mean of 10 months and after troglitazone withdrawal from the market, the patients were randomized to newer glitazones (rosiglitazone 4 mg and pioglitazone 30 mg). Seventy one patients with IGT or IR who received no antidiabetic medications served as control group. Patients were followed for a mean of 3 years in which patients treated with TZDs had a 88.9% risk reduction in progressing to diabetes compared to the control group.

In the ongoing DREAM study, 5269 patients with IGT, IFG or both were randomized to rosiglitazone and ramipril in a 2-by-2 factorial design in order to evaluate if rosiglitazone, ramipril or both reduces the incidence of diabetes and atherosclerosis [35]. This large study will give us valuable information concerning diabetes and cardiovascular prevention with TZDs and angiotension converting enzyme inhibitors (ACE inh).

Although TZD therapy appears to be promising in the prevention of type 2 diabetes, the only presently available data concerning prevention or delay of type 2 DM in RCT trials was obtained with metformin and acarbose therapy.

Prevention of Type 2 Diabetes in Patients Treated with Weight Loss Medications

In the Xenical in the Prevention of Diabetes in Obese Subjects (XENDOS) study [36], 3,305 obese patients (BMI $\geq$ 30 kg/m^2) were randomized to xenical therapy (120mg) or placebo three times daily and followed for 4 years. Mean weight loss after 4 years was 5.8 kg vs. 3.0 kg in the orlistat and placebo group respectively. The cumulative incidence of diabetes in the placebo group was 9.0% while in the orlistat group it was 6%, corresponding to a risk reduction of 37.3%. The protective effect of orlistat was observed only in the subgroup with IGT, and in this group there was a 41% risk reduction in progression to diabetes. In the group of patients with normal glucose tolerance (NGT), the incidence of diabetes was very low (2.7% over 4 years) and not statistically significant as compared to the orlistat treated patients (2.6% over 4 years).

Prevention of Type 2 Diabetes Mellitus with ACE Inhibitors or Angiotensin II Type 1 Receptor Blockers (ARB)

The renin-angiotensin system (RAS) controls fluid and electrolyte balance, and its main effector angiotension II (Ang II) has also inflammatory properties [37]. It is well known that blocking the RAS system through inhibition of Ang II formation or blockage of its receptor (angiotensin II 1 receptor- AT_1) is known to reduce morbidity and mortality associated with cardiovascular and kidney disease, particularly in diabetic patients [38].

ACE inhibitors and ARBs have been extensively studied in patients with hypertension, coronary heart disease and congestive heart failure. The effect of these drugs in diabetes prevention has been evaluated as secondary sub-group analysis or *post hoc* analysis.

Recently, Gillespie *et al* [39] published a meta-analysis including 11 randomized clinical trial and a total of 66,608 patients, evaluating the impact of ACE inhibitors and ARBs in the prevention of type 2 DM. Six trials evaluated the effect of ACE inhibitors [40-45] and 5 trials the effect of ARBs [46-50]. ACE inhibitors and ARB therapy significantly reduced the development of new onset type 2 diabetes whether patients had hypertension, coronary heart disease or chronic heart failure (IR 0.78 [95% CI 0.73-0.83]) [39]. Possible mechanisms involved in diabetes prevention in patients treated with ACE inhibitors and ARBs include an improvement in insulin sensitivity and an improvement in glucose tolerance [51].

The effect of ACE inhibitors and ARBs in the prevention of type 2 DM and cardiovascular disease as primary outcome are presently being evaluated in the DREAM study (rosiglitazone and ramipril) and in the NAVIGATOR trial (nateglinide and valsartan)[35,52]. The result of these 2 prospective studies including more than 8000 patients will possibly clarify the effect of ACE inh and ARB therapy in diabetes prevention.

Bariatric Surgery for the Prevention of Type 2 Diabetes Mellitus

At present, bariatric surgery is the most effective method to achieve appreciable, long term weight loss. Bariatric surgery reduces body weight by 35-40% with long-term maintenance of weight loss [53]. Weight loss is well known to improve obesity-related comorbidities including diabetes, hypertension and hyperlipidemia among many others.

Weight loss is promoted by gastric restriction and intestinal malabsorption (intestinal malaborption is obtained in patients that had the Roux-en-Y gastric bypass (RYGB)). Changes in body weight and glucose homeostasis are more pronounced in patients that had RYGB procedure. It seems that intestinal hormones are involved in the decreased appetite reported in patients undergoing bariatric surgery. Ghrelin levels are reported to be decreased in patients who had undergone bariatric surgery [54], partly explaining the decreased appetite reported in these patients. It is possible that increased delivery of nutrients to the hindgut promotes secretion of peptide YY (PYY) and glucagon-like peptide 1 (GLP-1), decreasing food intake and improving glucose tolerance [53,55] Numerous studies have shown complete remission of diabetes in approximately 83% of patients that had bariatric surgery. The prospective, controlled Swedish Obese Subjects Study, included patients who had gastric surgery and matched conventionally treated obese subjects. A report of patients enrolled for 2 years (4047 patients) or 10 years (1703 patients) showed a lower incidence of diabetes in the surgical group compared to the control group. The incidence of diabetes was 1% in the surgical group followed for 2 years compared to 8% in the control group (86% risk reduction). At 10 years the cumulative incidence of diabetes was 7% in the surgical group and 24% in the control group (5% risk reduction)[56].

Conclusion

There is now mounting evidence that type 2 DM can be prevented or delayed. Lifestyle changes including weight loss and an increase in physical activity have been shown to be highly effective in preventing type 2 diabetes in patients with IGT. The intensive programs used in recently published clinical trials may be too costly for national implementation but moderate weight loss (5-10% of body weight) in overweight and obese individuals and modest physical activity (30 min daily) should be recommended to all adults, particularly in high risk patients.

Pharmacotherapy has also shown to be effective in the prevention of type 2DM, but they have not been yet implemented in clinical practice possibly due to cost-effectiveness. Undergoing studies will shed more light on the role of pharmacotherapy in diabetes prevention.

Bariatric surgery has been shown to be highly effective in diabetes prevention for patients having surgery due to morbid obesity, but cannot be implemented as a population strategy.

References

[1]   Engelgau MM, Geiss LS, Saadine JB, Boyle JP, Benjamin SM, Gregg EW, et al (2004). The evolving diabetes burden in the United States. *Ann. Intern. Med*, 2004 140, 945-950.

[2]   King H, Aubert RE, Herman WH. Global burden of diabetes, 1995-2025: prevalence, numerical estimates, and projections. *Diabetes Care*, 1998, 21, 1414-1431.

[3]   Smyth S, Heron A.(2005) Diabetes and obesity: the twin epidemics. *Nature Medicine, 12*: 75-80.

[4]   Kuczmarski RJ, Flegal KM, Campbell SM, Johnson CL.Increasing prevalence of overweight among US adults. The National Health and Nutrition Examination Surveys 1960 to 1991. *JAMA*, 1994,272, 205-211.

[5]   Mokdad AH, Serdula MK, Dietz WH, Bowman BA, Marks JS, Koplan JP.The spread of the obesity epidemic in the United States. *JAMA*, 2001; 286: 1195-1200.

[6]   Leong KS, Wilding JP.Obesity and diabetes. *Baillieres Best Pract. Res. Clin. Endocrinol. Metab*.1999, 13; 221-237.

[7]   Fong DS, Aiello LP, Ferris GL 3rd, Klein R.Diabetic Retinopathy. *Diabetes Care*, 2004; 27: 2540-2553.

[8]   Boulton AJ, Vileikyte L, Ragnarson-Tennvall G, Apelqvist J.The global burden of diabetic food disease. *Lancet*, 2005; 12: 1719-1724.

[9]   DeFronzo RA & Ferranini E.Insulin resistance: a multifaceted syndrome responsible for NIDDM, obesity, hypetension, dyslipidemia, and atherosclerotic cardiovascular disease. *Diabetes Care*, 1991; 14:173-194.

[10] Turner RE, Millns H, Neil HA, Stratton IM, Manley SE, Matthews DR, Holman RR.Risk factors for coronary artery disease in non-insulin dependent diabetes mellitus: United Kingdom Prospective Diabetes Study (UKPDS 23). *BMJ*, 1998; 316:823-828.

[11] The Diabetes Control and Complications Trial Research Group.The effect of intensive treatment of diabetes on the development and progression of long-term complications in insulin-dependent diabetes mellitus. *N. Engl. J. Med*, 1993; 329:977-986.

[12] UK Prospective Diabetes Study (UKPDS) Group.Intensive blood-glucose control with sulphonylureas or insulin compared with conventional treatment and rik of complications in patients with type 2 diabetes (UKPDS 33). *Lancet*, 1998; 352: 837-853.

[13] UK Prospective Diabetes Study (UKPDS) Group.Effect of intensive blood-glucose control with metformin on complications in overweight patients with type 2 diabetes (UKPDS 34). *Lancet*, 1998; 352:854-865.

[14] Position statement. Diagnosis and classification of diabetes mellitus. *Diabetes Care*, 2006; 29: S43-48.

[15] Shaw JE, Zimmet PZ, de Courten M, Dowse GK, Chitsone P, Gareeboo H, Hemraj F et al.(1999). Impaired fasting glucose or impaired glucose tolerance. What best predicts future diabetes in Mauritius? *Diabetes Care*, 1999; 22: 399-402.

[16] Petersen JL, McGuire DK. Imapaired glucose tolerance and impaired fasting glucose- a review of diagnosis, clinical implications and management. *Diab. Vasc. Dis. Res*, 2005;1: 9-15.

[17] Saydah SH, Loria CM, Eberhardt MS, Brancati FL. Subclinical stages of glucose intolerance and risk of death in the US. *Diabetes Care*, 2001;24: 447-453.

[18] Eastman RC, Cowie CC, Harris MI: Undiagnosed diabetes or impaired glucose tolerance and cardiovascular risk. *Diabetes Care*, 1997; 20: 127-128.

[19] The DECODE Study Group: Glucose tolerance and cardiovascular mortality: comparison of fasting and 2 hour diagnostic criteria. *Arch. Intern. Med*, 2001;161: 397-405.

[20] Grundy S,Cleeman JI, Daniels SR, Donato KA, Eckel RH, Franklin BA, et al. Diagnosis and management of the metabolic syndrome. *Circulation*, 2005; 112: 2735-2752.

[21] Ford ES, Giles WH, Mokdad AH. Increasing prevalenc of the metabolic syndrome among U.S. adults. *Diabetes Care*, 2004; 27: 2444-2449.

[22] Pan XR, Li GW, Hu YH, Wang JX, Yang WY, An ZX et al. Effects of diet and exercise in preventing NIDDM in people with impaired glucose tolerance. The Da Qing IGT and Diabetes Study. *Diabetes Care*, 1997; 20: 537-544.

[23] Tuomilehto J, Lindstrom J, Eriksson JG, Valle TT, Hamalainen H, Ilanne-Parikka P et al. Prevention of type 2 diabetes mellitus by changes in lifestyle among subjects with impaired glucose tolerance. *N. Engl. J. Med*, 2001; 344: 1343-1350.

[24] Diabetes Prevention Program Research Group. Reduction in the incidence of type 2 diabetes with lifestyle intervention or metformin. *N. Engl. J. Med*, 2002; 346: 393-403.

[25] Orchard TJ, Temprosa M, Goldberg R, Haffner S, Ratner R, Marovina S, Fowler S for Diabetes Prevention Program Research Group. The effect of metformin and intensive lifestyle intervention on the metabolic syndrome: The Diabetes Prevention Program. *Inter. Med*, 2005; 142: 611-619.

[26] Curtis J, Wilson C. Preventing type 2 diabetes mellitus. *J. Am. Board. Fam. Pract*, 2005; 18: 37-43.

[27] The Diabetes Prevention Program Research Group: Effects of withdrawal from metformin on the development of diabetes in the Diabetes Prevention Program. *Diabetes Care*, 26: 977-980, 2003.

[28] Chiasson JL, Josse RG, Gomis R, Hanefeld , Karasik A, Markku Laakso. Acarbose for prenvention of type 2 diabetes mellitus: the STOP-NIDDM randomized trial. *Lancet*, 2002; 359: 2072-2077.

[29] Chiasson JL, Josse RG, Gomis R, Hanefeld M, karaik A, Laakso M: Acarbose treatment and the risk of cardiovascular disease and hypertension in patient with impaired glucose tolerance: the STOP-NIDDM trial. *JAMA*, 290: 486-494, 20003.

[30] Kendall DM. Thiazolidinediones- the case for early use. *Diabetes Care*, 2006; 29: 154-157.

[31] Staels B, Fruchart JC. Therapeutic roles of peroxisome proliferator-activated receptor agonists. *Diabetes*, 2005; 54: 2460-2470.

[32] Tan MH, Baksi A, Krahulec B, Kubalski P, Stankiewicz A, Urquhart R, Edwards G, Johns D, the GLAL Study Group: Comparison of pioglitazone and glicazide in sustaining glycemic control over 2 years in patients with type 2 diabetes. *Diabetes Care*, 28: 544-550, 2005.

[33] Buchanan TA, Xiang AH, Peters RK, Kjos SL, Marroquin A, Goico J, Ochoa C, Tan S, Berkoviwitz K, Hodis HN, Azen SP. Preservation of pancreatic β-cell function and prevention of type 2 diabetes by pharmacological treatment of insulin resistance in high-risk Hispanic women. *Diabetes*, 2002; 51: 2796-2803.

[34] The diabetes Prevention Program Research Program. Prevention of Type 2 diabetes with troglitazone in the Diabetes Prevention Program. *Diabetes*, 54:1150-1156, 2005.

[35] Durbin RJ. Thiazolidinedione therapy in the prevention/delay of type 2 diabetes in patients with impaired glucose tolerance and insulin resistance. *Diabetes, Obesity and Metabolism*, 2004, 280-285.

[36] Gerstein HC, Yusuf S, Holman R, The DREAM Trial Investigators. Rationale, design and recruitment characteristics of a large, simple international trial of diabetes prevention: the DREAM trial. *Diabetologia*, 2004 ; 47: 1519-1527.

[37] Torgerson JS, Hauptman J, Bodrin MN, Sjostrom L. Xenical in the prevention of diabetes in obese subjects. *Diabetes Care*, 27: 155-161,2004.

[38] Sironi L, Nobili E, Gianella A, Gelosa P, Tremoli E. Anti-inflammatory properties of drugs acting on the rennin-angiotensin system. *Drugs today (Barc,)* 2005; 41: 609-622.

[39] Podar T, Tuomilehto J. The role of angiotensin converting enzyme inhibitors and angiotensin II receptor antagonists in the management of diabetic complications. *Drugs*, 2002; 62: 2007-2012.

[40] Gillespie EL, White CM, Kardas M, Lindberg M and Coleman CI. The impact of ACE inhibitors or angiotensin II type 1 receptor blockers on the development of new-onset type 2 diabetes. *Diabetes Care*, 2005; 28:2261-2266.

[41] Hansson L, Lindholm LH, Ekbom T, Dahlof B, Schersten B, Wester PO, Hedner T, Faire UD: Randomised trial of old and new antihypertensive drugs in elderly patients: cardiovascular mortality and morbidity the Swedish trial in old patients with hypertension-2 study. *Lancet*, 1999; 354:1751–1756

[42] Hansson L, Lindholm LH, Niskanen L, Lanke J, Hedner T, Niklason A, Luomanmaki K, Dahlof B, Faire UD, Morlin C, Karlberg BE, Wester PO, Bjorck JE: Effect of angiotensin-converting-enzyme inhibition compared with conventional therapy on

cardiovascular morbidity and mortaility in hypertension: the captopril prevention project (CAPPP) randomized trial. *Lancet*, 1999; 353:611–616.

[43] ALLHAT Officers and Coordinators for the ALLHAT Collaborative Research Group, the Antihypertensive and Lipid-Lowering Treatment to Prevent Heart Attack Trial: Major outcomes in high-risk hypertensive patients randomized to angiotensin-converting enzyme inhibitor or calcium channel blocker vs diuretic: the antihypertensive and lipid-lowering treatment to prevent heart attack trail (ALLHAT). *JAMA*, 2002; 288:2981–2997.

[44] Braunwald E, Domanski MJ, Fowler SE, Geller NL, Gersh BJ, Hsia J, Pfeffer MA, Rice MM, Rosenberg YD, Rouleau JL, the PEACE Trial Investigators: Angiotensin-converting-enzyme inhibition in stable coronary artery disease. *N. Engl. J. Med*, 2004; 351:2058–2068.

[45] Yusuf S, Sleight P, Pogue J, Bosch J, Davies R, Dagenais G: Effects of an angiotensin-converting-enzyme inhibitor, ramipril, on cardiovascular events in high-risk patients: the Heart Outcomes Prevention Evulation Study Investigators. *N Engl J Med*, 2000; 342:145–153.

[46] Wing LMH, Ried CM, Ryan P, Beilin LJ, Brown MA, Jennings GLR, Johnston CI, McNeil JJ, Macdonald GJ, Marley JE, Morgan TO, West MJ: A comparison of outcomes with angiotensin-converting-enzyme inhibitors and diuretics for hypertension in the elderly. *N. Engl. J. Med*, 2003; 348:583–592.

[47] Julius S, Kjeldsen SE, Weber M, Brunner HR, Ekman S, Hansson L, Hua T, Laragh J, McInnes GT, Mitchell L, Plat F, Schork A, Smith B, Zanchetti A: Outcomes in hypertensive patients at high cardiovascular risk treated with regimens based on valsartan or amlodipine: the VALUE randomized trial. *Lancet*, 2004; 363:2022–2031.

[48] Yusuf S, Pfeffer MA, Swedberg K, Granger CB, Held P, McMurray JJV, Michelson EL, Olofsson B, Ostergen J: Effects of candasartan in patients with chronic heart failure and preserved left-ventricular ejection fraction: the CHARM-Preserved trial. *Lancet,* 2003; 362:777–781.

[49] Granger CB, McMurray JJV, Yusuf S, Held P, Michelson EL, Olofsson B, Ostergeren J, Pfeffer MA, Swedberg K: Effects of candesartan in patients with chronic heart failure and reduced left-ventricular systolic function intolerant to angiotensin-converting-enzyme inhibitors: the CHARM-Alternative trial. *Lancet*, 2003; 362:772–776.

[50] Dahlof B, Devereux RB, Kjeelsen SE, Julius S, Beevers G, Faire UD, Fyhrquist F, Ibsen H, Kristiansson K, Lederballe-Pedersen O, Lindholm LH, Nieminen MS, Omvik P, Oparil S, Wedel H: Cardiovascular morbidity and mortality in the losaratan intervention for endpoint reduction in hypertension study (LIFE): a randomized trail against atenolol. *Lancet*, 2002;359:995–1003.

[51] Lithell H, Hansson L, Skoog I, Elmfeldt D, Hofman A, Olofsson B, Trenkwalder P, Zanchetti A: The study on cognition and prognosis in the elderly (SCOPE): principal results of a randomized double-blind intervention trial. *J. Hypertens*, 2003; 21:875–886.

[52] Ferrannini E, Seghieri G, Muscelli E. Insulin and the renin-angiotensin-aldosterone system: influence of ACE inhibition. *J. Cardiovasc. Pharmacol*, 1994; 24 Suppl. 3: S61-69.

[53] Nateglinide and valsartan in impaired glucose tolerance outcomes research: rationale and design of the NAVIGATOR trial. *Diabetes* 2002; 51 (Suppl. 2): A116.

[54] Cummings DE, Overduin J, Foster-Schubert KE. Gastric bypass for obesity: mechanisms of weight loss and diabetes resolution. *J. Clin. End. Metab.* 2004; 89: 2608-2615.

[55] Cummings DE, Weigle DS, Frayo RS, Breen PA, Ma MK, Dellinger EP, Purnell JG. Human plasma ghrelin levels after diet –induced weight loss and gastric bypass surgery. *N. Engl. J. Med*, 2002; 346: 1623-1630.

[56] Hickey M.S., Pories W.J., McDonals K.J. Jr, et al.A new paradign for type 2 diabetes mellitus: could it be a disease of the foregut? *Ann Surg*, 1998; 227, 637-643.

[57] Sjostrom L, Lindroos AK, Peltonen M, Trogerson J, Bouchard C, Carlsson B et al. Lifestyle, diabetes and cardiovascular risk factors 10 years after bariatric surgery. *N. Engl. J. Med*, 2004; 351: 2683-2693.

In: Progress in Metabolic Syndrome Research
Editor: George T. Ulrig, pp. 89-109

ISBN 1-60021-179-8
© 2006 Nova Science Publishers, Inc.

Chapter IV

The Emerging Role of Inflammatory Markers in the Metabolic Syndrome

Ali A. Rizvi[*]

Division of Endocrinology, Diabetes, and Metabolism,
University of South Carolina, School of Medicine,
Columbia, SC 29203 USA.

Abstract

The metabolic syndrome consists of a constellation of risk factors including obesity, glucose intolerance, hypertension, and dyslipidemia in the setting of insulin resistance that confers an increased risk of cardiovascular disease and type 2 diabetes. Although the major pathophysiologic mechanisms are still in the process of being elucidated, the possible role of inflammation, cytokines, and atherogenic markers has received attention lately. Recent studies suggest that inflammatory markers like C-reactive protein (CRP), Interleukin (IL)-6, and Tumor Necrosis Factor (TNF)-α mirror oxidative stress and may be instrumental in the final pathway of adverse vascular outcomes in the metabolic syndrome. Other adipocytokines produced by fatty tissue are also altered, with lower levels of adiponectin and increased leptin and resistin. Elevated Plasminogen Activator Inhibitor (PAI)-1 and fibrinogen levels, and derangement in clotting factors correlate with the degree of insulin resistance and may contribute to the prothrombotic tendency. Taken together, these abnormalities shift the balance of endothelial function towards an abnormal state that heightens the risk of atherothrombosis. Lifestyle factors and medications can have a profound effect in modifying these parameters. The phenomenal increase in the prevalence of obesity has accentuated the various clinical manifestations and pathopysiologic underpinnings of this epidemic. Continued research looking at the role of inflammation and cytokines in the genesis and propagation of the metabolic

[*] Correspondence concerning this article should be addressed to Ali A. Rizvi, MD, FACP, Associate Professor of Medicine, Division of Endocrinology, Diabetes, and Metabolism, University of South Carolina School of Medicine, Two Medical Park, Suite 502, Columbia, SC 29203, USA. Ph: 803-540-1000; Fax: 803-540-1050; Email: arizvi@gw.mp.sc.edu.

syndrome should provide a window into its pathogenesis at the cellular and humoral level, improve the understanding of disease mechanisms, and open up possibilities for effective therapeutic interventions in the future.

Keywords: metabolic syndrome, inflammation, C-reactive protein, adipocytokines, insulin resistance

Introduction: Vascular Inflammation, Metabolic Syndrome, Insulin Resistance, and Atherosclerosis

The prevalence of the metabolic syndrome or insulin resistance syndrome is increasing because of global changes in obesity, sedentary lifestyle, and the ageing of the population [1]. This syndrome consists of a clustering of cardiovascular risk factors in the setting of increased body weight (indicated mainly by increased waist circumference and body mass index or BMI). Insulin resistance is believed to play a major role in the underlying pathophysiology of the metabolic syndrome, contributing to atherosclerosis and increasing the risk of glucose intolerance and diabetes [2]. Thus a process of chronic and incremental damage to the arterial wall is begun that eventually leads to vascular complications. The resultant adverse cardiovascular events are usually clinically evident and well recognized. The various stages of the atherosclerotic process have been delineated [3], and have their origins in insults to the endothelium from a combination of factors. These predisposing conditions include the well-known risk factors, including hypertension, hyperlipidemia, hyperglycemia, and smoking [4]. Sustained noxious stimuli interact over time to damage the vascular integrity and shift the balance of the endothelial milieu towards one that promotes injury and progressive failure of repair mechanisms [5]. Chemotaxis of mononuclear cells ensues, leading to their adhesion, migration, and differentiation within the vessel wall. Deposition of lipids within the macrophages is favored by the availability of easily oxidizable lipoproteins. Meanwhile, migration and proliferation of smooth muscle cells into the intima forms a fibrous cap over this "fatty streak" and leads to the appearance of an atherosclerotic lesion [6]. At some point during its subsequent progression, the altered pathology predisposes to the formation of a thrombus, usually initiated by plaque rupture. Indeed, vulnerable plaques have been identified that seem to have distinctive morphological composition and are prone to rupture [7]. The end-result is a vascular event that can have catastrophic consequences.

It is generally agreed that a heightened, proinflammatory picture precedes and perpetuates the atherosclerotic process [8]. There may be an increased genetic susceptibility to oxidative stress that lays the groundwork for ongoing damage [9]. Insulin resistance has been implicated in not only accelerating the inflammation [10], but also being the ultimate catalyst for glucose intolerance, dyslipidemia, and hypertensive damage. The picture, however, is complicated and controversial. The "insulin resistance hypothesis" contends that an inability to satisfactorily maintain insulin-mediated glucose uptake into tissues has a broad array of deleterious ramifications, some of which can be directly linked to the resultant hyperinsulinemia [11]. However, both the NCEP ATP III and the IDF criteria for the diagnosis of the metabolic syndrome are based on clinical and laboratory measurements and are devoid of the need for direct computation of insulin resistance [12,13]. What is established is the unequivocal importance of these criteria as risk factors for cardiovascular disease and type 2 diabetes. Therefore, the central role of insulin resistance in a definition of the metabolic syndrome meant for use in clinical practice is unclear. In addition, weight gain and obesity will increase both inflammation and insulin resistance [14]. In fact, in some studies, the bulk of association between the two can be explained on the basis of increased body weight alone [15]. However, not all obese individuals are insulin-resistant or display a proinflammatory picture. In short, although the metabolic syndrome had its origins as the "insulin resistance syndrome" and is still preferred to be called by that name by some people, the part that insulin resistance itself plays in its causation and sequelae is yet to be fully defined. On the other hand, a wealth of evidence is accumulating regarding the connection between markers of inflammation and the clinically-defined 'metabolic syndrome' [16,17].

Inflammatory Markers as "Non-traditional" Risk Factors in the Metabolic Syndrome and Related Conditions

Inflammation is regarded as a contributor to morbidity in the closely related conditions of cardiovascular disease, obesity, the metabolic syndrome, and type 2 diabetes and has been the focus of extensive research recently [18,19]. Inflammatory markers like C-reactive protein (CRP), fibrinogen, the interleukins, tumor necrosis factor-alpha (TNF-α), tissue-type plasminogen activator, and serum amyloid A (SAA) have been included in the ever-expanding list of emerging or "non-traditional" risk factors for the atherosclerotic process [20] (figure 1). They mirror oxidative stress and generation of free radicals that can promote vascular damage, endothelial injury, plaque rupture, and athero-thrombosis [21]. Studies have established a significant inflammatory component in the background of clinically recognizable risk factors (for example, hypertension, hyperglycemia, dyslipidemia, obesity, and smoking) [22]. Inflammatory proteins like CRP have been shown to predict, and correlate independently with, major cardiovascular end-points like myocardial infarction and death [23,24].

Hypercoagulability states and hemostatic factors like fibrinogen have been postulated to play a pathologic role in the development of vascular complications, ostensibly through abnormal rheology and elevated blood viscosity [25,26]. Prospective studies show that low-grade systemic inflammation is associated with not only the development of diabetes, but also its large-vessel and microvascular complications [27,28,29]. Retinopathy and nephropathy are linked to increased levels of inflammatory markers in both type 1 and type 2 diabetes [30,31]. However, it is not clear if CRP measurement in diabetes and the metabolic syndrome provides added information beyond that obtained through the established risk factors. Increased body mass index (BMI) with or without the presence of the metabolic syndrome or diabetes, accounted for the bulk of the pro-inflammatory picture in some analyses [28]. The effect of race on variation in inflammatory markers has also been noted in Caucasians and African-Americans [32]. Therefore, more research is needed before screening can be advocated [32,33].

Since cardiovascular disease (CVD) and the metabolic syndrome are closely linked, any discussion of cardiac risk factors must necessarily overlap with the criteria designated for the metabolic syndrome. The traditional risk factors for CVD – positive family history, hypertension, diabetes, dyslipidemia, and smoking – explain a preponderant amount of morbidity and mortality, especially when combined with abdominal obesity, sedentary lifestyle, and diet composition. However, these traditional or established factors do not fully account for the CVD burden in certain populations (for example, those with diabetes) [34,35]. Attention has been focused recently on whether the "nontraditional" risk factors are independently associated with vascular risk, and if they provide clinically significant prognostic value beyond the established ones [35,36]. Interestingly, these emerging factors are almost exclusively circulating markers, and tend to cluster together among themselves and with the traditional factors [37]. Examples of these markers that have been studied in some detail include CRP, fibrinogen, the adipocytokines, and the proinflammatory cytokines. Several epidemiologic studies demonstrate that CRP is a reliable predictor of future cardiovascular events in individuals free of disease at baseline [23,24]. However, three important questions remain to be answered in the analysis of these new risk factors vis-à-vis coronary disease: firstly, since these parameters are acute-phase reactants that segregate with the traditional risk factors, do they confer some measure of independent risk or merely reflect what can already be gleaned from known information? Second, are they simply markers or do they represent true mediators of the underlying extent of inflammation? Some argue that they are simply epiphenomena with little direct pathogenetic role in disease causation. However, the inherent proinflammatory actions of some of these markers point to a possible etiologic and pathologic implication in the disease process. Finally, it is not yet clear if clinical management can be altered on the basis of screening for these emerging factors. The answer to this last question is predicated on whether a treatment is developed that directly targets the various inflammatory markers without altering the established risk factors and subsequently evaluating clinical outcomes.

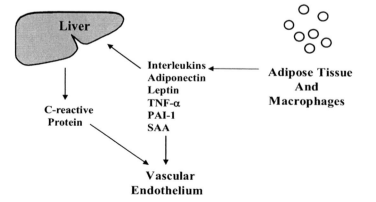

Figure 1. Interactions between adipose tissue, liver, and the vascular endothelium by way of the inflammatory markers and cytokines.

C-reactive Protein

CRP is the best-known marker of inflammation and has been touted as an independent risk factor for cardiovascular disease on the basis of recent studies. It is a member of the pentraxin family, which consists of five noncovalently associated peptides surrounding a central core. It is an acute-phase reactant that is synthesized in the liver and activates the classical pathway of complement through the immune system. Various proinflammatory cytokines such as tumor necrosis factor and interleukin-1 derived from vascular endothelium and adipose tissue stimulate its formation. The release of interleukin-6 from macrophages by increased oxidative stress and infection may be the original insult that initiates this process. CRP has been shown to tilt the balance of endovascular health towards a proatherogenic state by reducing the synthesis and biological activity of nitric oxide, upregulating endothelin-1, and activating cell adhesion molecules.

Numerous studies have revealed that persons that have the most or all features of the metabolic syndrome have increased levels of CRP [38,39,40]. It has been linked to insulin resistance, dyslipidemic states, blood pressure, and increased amounts of other proinflammatory cytokines [41]. The Insulin Resistance and Atherosclerosis Study showed that CRP values correlated with body mass index (BMI), waist circumference, and fasting hyperinsulinemia [42]. There is a linear correlation between CRP and the number of metabolic abnormalities present, namely upper-body obesity, dyslipidemia, hyperglycemic states, and hypertension [43]. For all levels of glucose, the presence of metabolic syndrome was associated with an increase in the prevalence of CVD [44]. The metabolic syndrome appears to be associated with inflammation in addition to being an important marker of CVD risk. CVD prevalence is greater in persons with metabolic syndrome without diabetes than in those with diabetes who do not have the metabolic syndrome [45]. CRP levels in nondiabetic persons increase with worsening glycemia and particularly with postload glycemia [46,47]. The Third National Health and Nutrition Examination Survey (NHANES III) data confirmed that subjects with the metabolic syndrome were more likely to have higher levels of CRP and other markers of inflammation [45]. Based on Framingham scores, CRP adds prognostic information to the predictive power of other CVD risk factors like cholesterol, hypertension, and cigarette use [20]. It confers a stronger predisposition to CVD than other known inflammatory markers such as homocysteine, IL-6, and SAA, circulating levels of which parallel CRP, intracellular adhesion molecule-1 (ICAM)-I [48,49], as well as low-density lipoprotein (LDL), the time-honored correlate of cardiovascular risk [50]. Obese persons have improvement in insulin sensitivity and in CRP with weight loss. On the other hand, obese persons with normal insulin sensitivity with low CRP levels do not show further decrease following weight loss. This suggests that improvement in insulin sensitivity rather than weight loss mediates the reduction in CRP [51].

The reasons for the discrepant results regarding the benefit of using CRP in evaluating risk are not known. Possible explanations include different sets of populations studied, and their retrospective versus prospective nature. CRP, as well as other inflammatory markers, is acutely elevated in stress, illnesses, infections, and vascular events like myocardial infarction and unstable angina. CRP appears to be of greatest use in risk assessment of persons who have intermediate CVD risk (10-20%/10 years) [22]. Insulin resistance is associated with increased CRP levels, and in some studies CRP has been found to be an independent CVD risk factor [52-56]and a marker of insulin resistance [57-60]. Three studies examined the relationship between CRP, the metabolic syndrome, and incident cardiovascular events [57,61,62]. In these large population studies, CRP was a strong independent predictor of events, and its predictive value was equal to that of the metabolic syndrome. In two studies [55,61] the age-adjusted relative risk of future events was the same in subjects with high CRP without the metabolic syndrome and in subjects with low CRP with the metabolic syndrome. Interestingly, in subjects with both elevated CRP levels and the presence of the metabolic syndrome, the relative risk of events was double than in the other subgroups. This indicates that CRP measurement might have extra predictive power when added to the clinical definition of the metabolic syndrome. Rutter et al. [62] also found that CRP and the metabolic syndrome were independent risk factors, but in contrast to the two other reports, combining CRP and metabolic syndrome did not improve the predictive value of either used alone. Reilly et al. [63] also found that CRP did not add significantly to the metabolic syndrome, but their study did not include CVD outcomes.

Adiponectin

Our understanding of the functions of the adipose tissue has changed significantly with research suggesting that it not merely an inert storage site for excess energy. Instead, fatty tissue appears to be hormonally active and gives rise to a number of biologically active substances that regulate, and correlate with, insulin sensitivity, vascular function, and atherosclerotic disease. Collectively known as "adipocytokines", these molecules include, but are not limited to, adiponectin, leptin, resistin, IL-6, TNF-α, and plasminogen activator inhibitor-1 (PAI-1). An emerging concept is that obesity leads to infiltration of adipose tissues by macrophages which produce most of the inflammatory cytokines that are commonly measured [19] and contribute to insulin resistance. In addition, both macrophages and adipose tissue cells are thought to produce factors like IL-6 that secondarily increase hepatic CRP synthesis. Overfeeding may lead to a state of chronic macrophage activation, increased cytokines, central obesity, insulin resistance, and overproduction of the hepatic products of cytokine activation.

Adiponectin is produced by fat cells, and has properties that inhibit inflammation and enhance insulin sensitivity. It increases glucose transport and fatty acid oxidation. In animal studies, a deficiency of this cytokine can permit changes in metabolism to take place that favor the development of a metabolic syndrome phenotype [64]. It has been shown to suppress endothelial dysfunction, lipid accumulation, smooth muscle proliferation, and inhibit atherosclerotic changes in vessel walls. Low levels of adiponectin are found in subjects with diabetes and obesity, and correlate with insulin resistance and the future development of glucose intolerance and the metabolic syndrome. It has anti-inflammatory and antiatherogenic properties at the molecular level, such as decreasing the expression of adhesion molecules, reducing monocyte adhesion to endothelial cells, and suppressing various proatherogeic steps, such as uptake of oxidized LDL, foam cell formation, and proliferation and migration of vascular smooth muscle cells [65]. Other effects include increased insulin sensitivity and free fatty-acid oxidation oxidation, and decreased hepatic glucose production, and intracellular triglycerides. Adiponectin levels are lower in obesity and in prediabetes, and persons with higher levels of adiponectin have greater insulin sensitivity regardless of weight [66].

The question of whether a better understanding of the relationship between adiponectin and inflammation will lead to new or improved ways of addressing the metabolic syndrome is still unresolved. The connection between adiponectin and the clinical correlates of the metabolic syndrome is complex. It is interesting that obesity by itself in not necessarily associated with hypoleptinemia. Visceral obesity is predominantly associated with reduced levels of adiponectin. Obese women who have normal amounts of upper-body adipose tissue have normal adiponectin levels [67]. Low adiponectin was predictive of an increased future risk of coronary thrombosis in the Health Professionals Follow-up Study (HPFS), even after controlling for age, body weight, blood pressure, glucose control, physical activity, and tobacco use [68]. There seems to be a close relationship between adiponectin and HDL cholesterol [67,68] and the predictive power of adiponectin can partly be explained on their co-segregation.

In summary, adiponectin is inversely associated with insulin resistance, inflammation, blood pressure, LDL cholesterol, HDL cholesterol, and triglyceride levels. Multiple studies have established a correlation between adiponectin and CVD [69-72] and low levels of this adipocytokine found in subjects with the clinical characteristics of the metabolic syndrome.

Other Adipocytokines and Inflammatory Markers

Other markers of inflammation, described in some detail below, correlate with both insulin resistance and hyperinsulinemia. Since they are also elevated in obesity and in the presence of cardiovascular risk factors [42], they provide further evidence towards the idea that inflammation is an integral part of the components of the metabolic syndrome. CRP, the most extensively studied inflammatory marker, is strongly associated with adipose-derived cytokines including interleukin-6 and TNF-α [73]. These are likely to be elevated in obese insulin-resistant subjects, especially in those with upper-body fat deposition, but not generally in obese subjects who are insulin-sensitive [51]. Since these markers have been linked to dyslipidemia, hypertension, and insulin levels [42,74], they have been implicated in the genesis and progression of CVD [7,17].

Interleukin-6 is a cytokine that is produced in part in the adipose tissue, especially omental fat. It is released in response to stress and stimulation through the sympathetic nervous system. Several studies suggest that it is a central mediator of the inflammatory response, and tends to correlates closely with CRP [75,76]. IL-6 is increased with increasing insulin resistance and in the presence of multiple features of the metabolic syndrome [77]. It increases hepatic triglyceride secretion and may be a factor in central obesity and insulin resistance. It seems to exert its metabolic actions both through its actions in the central nervous system (CNS) and on peripheral organs. Levels of IL-6 are linked to insulin resistance and adiposity [78]. Its exact pathogenetic in glucose and lipid homeostasis in human is still a matter of debate.

Tumor Necrosis Factor-α is produced by largely by adipose tissue, but also by macrophages and endothelial cells. Its levels correlate with amount of adipose tissue, and it has a role in modulating insulin sensitivity [79]. It has been linked to the increase in insulin resistance seen with obesity [80], although a consistent correlation of TNF-α with BMI has not been conclusively demonstrated. Although it has been implicated in states of increased insulin resistance, passive immunization with antibodies to TNF-α does not improve insulin sensitivity.

The discovery of *leptin* generated great interest when it was found to have a role in obesity, energy balance, and appetite regulation. Hypoleptinemia has been linked to weight gain, fat deposition in organs such as the liver, muscle, and pancreatic islets, clinical features of the metabolic syndrome, and a general proinflammatory state [81]. Leptin could have the property of lowering insulin levels. Resistance to leptin may be connected to the hyperinsulinemia that is the earliest compensatory defect in the pathway towards the metabolic syndrome and glucose intolerance. Efforts at harnessing the known properties of this hormone to therapeutic purposes have so far been unsuccessful.

Leptin is secreted by adipocytes and binds to receptors in the CNS, where it suppresses appetite and decreases food intake. In the peripheral tissues, it enhances insulin sensitivity in muscle and fatty tissue, while preventing fat storage in organs such as the liver and pancreas [82]. It functions as a signaling factor that keeps the CNS informed of the status of energy availability in the body, especially as it pertains to the adipose tissue. Weight gain and overfeeding increase leptin expression and secretion, while reduced food intake suppresses them [83]. Leptin deficient mice (*ob/ob* mice) manifest extreme obesity. In humans, typical obesity is associated with increased leptin levels, signifying underlying leptin resistance. Whether leptin-resistant individuals are, therefore, prone to becoming overweight or if obesity aggravates resistance to leptin action is not entirely clear. The metabolic syndrome is also associated with increased levels of leptin [84]. However, most of this elevation can probably be explained on the basis of the extra weight alone. Does insulin resistance and the presence of other features of the metabolic syndrome modulate leptin release, or are more apt to be present if leptin resistance is present, is the subject of future debate and research.

Additional research has unveiled another adipocyte-derived cytokine, *resistin,* that is elevated in obesity and impaired glucose tolerance. Its role in the genesis and pathophysiology of the metabolic syndrome, however, remains to be fully elucidated.

Finally, insulin resistance is associated with a number of other inflammatory markers that have generated interest, such as secretory phospholipase A2, e-selectin, ICAM-1, and SAA [17]. Most of these are acute-phase reactants, whose production in the liver is induced by the interleukins and TNF-α. SAA appears to be a "scavenger" apolipoprotein that is closely linked with high-density lipoprotein (HDL). t is involved in lipid transport in the circulation, accelerating cholesterol uptake from damaged tissues, and may also play a role in immune regulation. Increased levels SAA that are seen after myocardial infarction are associated with an elevated risk of a recurrent coronary event [84]. In short, it may have an integrative role in such seemingly diverse areas as inflammation, atherosclerosis, and immunity. Further research is essential to unraveling its exact place in the inflammatory cascade and the obesity-metabolic syndrome spectrum. It is safe to say that, based on results of research done thus far, the inflammatory cytokines are critical in affecting the balance of endothelial health;

obesity, insulin resistance, stress, presence of the metabolic syndrome components, and other acute or chronic insults tend to tilt the balance towards a more proinflammatory picture and lead an environment conducive to atherogenesis and thrombosis. Components of the metabolic syndrome as well as the syndrome itself are associated with various measures of inflammation. This inflammatory picture is low-grade but chronic, and is associated with an increased risk for cardiovascular disease and diabetes. It provides a putative pathogenetic mechanism for the increased risk of adverse vascular outcomes that are experienced by individuals with the metabolic syndrome.

Hypercoagulablity and Hemostasis in the Metabolic Syndrome

The metabolic syndrome has been found to be associated with increased levels of fibrinogen [85,86] enhanced platelet adhesion [87] and impaired fibrinolysis [88,89] and elevated PAI-1 [90]. The latter is probably the most consistent abnormality seen in persons with the metabolic syndrome. In addition, endothelial dysfunction is linked to increased levels of clotting factors like factor VIII and von Willibrand's factor [91]. These changes are closely associated with insulin resistance and cardiovascular risk factors. The overall effect is an increased tendency to clotting and thrombus formation, as well as a reduced capacity to mitigate the pro-thrombotic tendency from impaired fibrinolysis. An elevated risk of atherothrombosis and cardiovascular obstructive events ensues.

PAI-1 levels are strongly associated with dyslipidemia, hyperinsulinemia, and hypertension [92,93]. It is noteworthy that the effect of increased PAI-1 was mitigated to a nonsignificant level after adjusting for BMI and elevated triglycerides in one study [94] In the Cardiovascular Health Study [93] levels of procoagulant factors and vitamin K-dependent proteins were studied in association with the different components of the metabolic syndrome. PAI-1 stood out as having the most consistent correlation with body weight, hyperglycemia, and hyperinsulinemia. TNF-α and IL-6 have been shown to induce synthesis of fibrinogen in the liver. Additional evidence of the connection between insulin resistance and defective fibrinolysis is provided by the possible involvement of the renin-angiotensin system and abnormalities of platelet function. The former is activated in obese, insulin-resistant subjects, who have higher levels of angiotensinogen and increased PAI-1 formation and release. Increased platelet activation and aggregation is found in subjects with the metabolic syndrome and type 2 diabetes as well [87].

In summary, the metabolic syndrome is a hypercoagulable state that is a feature of the underlying insulin resistance. It predisposes to clot formation in the milieu of endothelial dysfunction, endovascular atheromatous change, and abnormal blood rheology. Studies to date have shown evidence for a pathophysiologic role of the inflammatory markers in promoting a prothrombotic tendency and impairing the ability of fibrinolytic repair and resumption of blood flow. However, many of the interconnections between the coagulation system, inflammation, and the individual risk factors of the metabolic syndrome have yet to be clearly delineated.

Metabolic Syndrome and Inflammation in the Pediatric Population

Although a wealth of information about the metabolic syndrome has accumulated in adults, research about the prevalence and manifestations of the syndrome among children and adolescents is limited. Preliminary studies reveal that, like their adult counterparts, children and adolescents with the metabolic syndrome are more likely than those without this syndrome to show evidence of low-grade inflammation and increased levels of proinflammatory cytokines.

The association between obesity and elevated concentrations of CRP in children and adolescents has been clearly established [95,96]. The percentage of children and adolescents with an elevated concentration of CRP (>3.0 mg/l) is manifold higher among those with the metabolic syndrome compared with those who did not have the syndrome. In these studies, visceral obesity was the component that was responsible for much of the difference in concentrations of CRP. Concentrations of CRP have also been significantly associated with the other four components of the metabolic syndrome [97,98]. However, after adjustment for an anthropometric measure, many of these associations were seriously weakened and often failed to achieve statistical significance. Although no studies have thus far shown that children and adolescents with evidence of low-grade inflammation are more likely to develop cardiovascular disease or diabetes than those without such evidence, obesity in childhood does increase the risk for diabetes in childhood and a variety of diseases in adulthood [99]. Results of a recent study suggest that the presence of the metabolic syndrome and abdominal obesity among children and adolescents may be lay the foundation for the emergence of cardiovascular disease and diabetes later in life through early low-grade inflammation [100]. To reduce the potential adverse effects of the inflammation that accompanies the metabolic syndrome, a concerted public health and behavioral approach is needed to reduce the burden of obesity and physical inactivity in children. This strategy will not only prevent the development of the syndrome and its attendant proinflammatory manifestations, but also ameliorate these features in those who already have the metabolic syndrome or its components

Effect of Various Interventions on Inflammatory Markers in the Metabolic Syndrome

The trio of the metabolic syndrome, cardiovascular disease, and increased inflammation has assumed enhanced priority because of their direct implication in fueling the epidemics of type 2 diabetes and vascular disease [17,101]. In the absence of any approved drug therapy, modulation of the inflammatory state by lifestyle factors in the metabolic syndrome assumes paramount importance [102]. This is even more significant in view of the fact that dietary factors and lack of physical activity in the modern-day world forms the basis for the enormous increase in the prevalence of the metabolic syndrome. It makes sense, therefore, to attack the very dynamics that contribute to the genesis of the syndrome. Attainment of an ideal body weight and normalization of BMI, preferably by a combination of physical activity and a calorie-restricted diet, form the cornerstone of therapeutic measures for the metabolic syndrome. Weight loss has been shown to reduce the inflammatory markers associated with insulin resistance. The composition of the diet is important as well – a Mediterranean-style diet rich in fruits, nuts, whole grains, and olive oil has been shown to have a beneficial effect on the metabolic syndrome and its clinical and inflammatory components [103]. Polyunsaturated, omega-3, and linoleic acid supplementation has also been shown to help [104]. Weight loss reduces the prevalence of steatohepatitis, an emerging facet of the metabolic syndrome that is closely associated with increased inflammatory markers [105]. Exercise has been shown to reduce the proinfammatory and prothrombotic picture in individuals who have the clinical criteria of the metabolic syndrome [106]. Sustained physical activity also has a salutary effect on chemokines and other mediators in insulin resistance [107]. The involvement of dieticians and other health care professionals is of vital importance in educating individuals of the need for dietary modifications in preventing the adverse sequelae of obesity and the metabolic syndrome [108]. Cigarette smoking has been shown to elevate proinflammatory markers as well as insulin resistance itself in a Japanese study [109].

There are no drugs that have been approved solely for the treatment of the metabolic syndrome or for targeting the heightened inflammatory state involved therein. At the time of writing, no guidelines recommend routine testing, targeting, or monitoring of CRP levels, the most extensively studies marker in states on insulin resistance. However, medication already in use for the treatment of metabolic conditions like diabetes, hypertension, and dyslipidemia have been shown to reduce inflammation in susceptible individuals through various mechanisms. A detailed description of the actions of these drugs on markers of inflammation is beyond the scope of this review. Perhaps the best known are the thiazolidinediaones, agents that directly ameliorate insulin resistance by acting on the peroxisome-proliferator activator receptor-gamma (PPAR-γ) nuclear receptors. Numerous studies have proven their efficacy in reducing markers of inflammation [110,111,112] and improving endothelial function and lipid profile and blood pressure. The two agents currently available on the market, rosiglitazone and pioglitazone, have both been studied in this respect. An unwanted side-effect, however, is the tendency to weight gain, fluid accumulation, and possible precipitation of overt congestive heart failure. Although this class of medications is widely used for the treatment of type 2 diabetes, it is not yet approved for use in prediabetes or the metabolic syndrome.

Several other medications have approved indications and target risk factors for cardiovascular disease as well as individual components of the metabolic syndrome. The HMG Co-A reductase inhibitors ("statins") are proven for their lipid-lowering properties and for reducing cardiac and all-cause mortality. Several large clinical trials showed that they decreased inflammatory markers, notably CRP levels, in high-risk individuals with dyslipidemia, diabetes, and the metabolic syndrome [55,113,114]. This action is part of their non-lipid-lowering, or pleotropic, efficacy on the vascular endothelium [115,116]. Fibric-acid derivatives have also been advocated as useful agents in counter-acting the elevated inflammatory milieu of the metabolic syndrome [117].

Two other therapeutic modalities appear to be beneficial in the metabolic syndrome by reducing the proinflammatory and thrombotic cascade: targeting the renin-angiotensin system through the use of angiotensin-converting enzyme inhibitors [118] and angiotensin-receptor blocking agents [119] and use of aspirin to decrease the primary as well as secondary incidence of coronary thrombosis in patients with existing cardiovascular disease or those with multiple risk factors [120]. Most individuals with the metabolic syndrome will satisfy the clinical requirement for use of these agents and it is plausible that a significant portion of their salutary mechanisms are mediated by means of their anti-inflammatory actions. Specifically targeting the inflammatory pathways and mediators in insulin resistance and the metabolic syndrome is still uncharted territory, though a promising next step, of future drug therapy [121,122].

The Inflammatory Markers as Screening Tools and Therapeutic Targets

There is currently no consensus in using the markers of inflammation as screening tools or as risk factors to be targeted. This area appears to be embroiled in controversy and confusion, although some recommendations have been put forth [8,9]. The argument for testing of individuals at moderate risk for cardiovascular disease is based on further stratifying their risk status and assist in clinical management. On the other hand, some contend that the role of these acute-phase reactants in disease causation is not established, and therefore screening would not be helpful in leading to a change in management strategy for the majority of patients tested. Additionally, the lack of specific and proven therapeutic interventions targeting these markers (beyond what is already being recommended) is also a factor against using them in routine clinical setting. Whether to include CRP or some other inflammatory marker in the clinical criteria used in the diagnosis of the metabolic syndrome is dependent upon elucidation of their exact role in the pathogenesis of the syndrome and their connection to underlying insulin resistance. In other words, the question of whether these markers are merely the mirror of a chronic vasculotoxic pattern or are causally involved in endothelial dysfunction and atherosclerosis is central from the viewpoint of using them for screening, assessment, and treatment in the metabolic syndrome and related conditions. Further research is needed to clarify the etiology of the metabolic syndrome at the molecular and inflammatory level and possibly to a definition that includes one or more of the inflammatory markers. Hopefully, a new model of the metabolic syndrome can be validated so that its predictive value is inclusive of clinical as well as laboratory criteria. Additional studies concerning the markers of inflammation, ideally performed in a prospective, randomized, and interventional manner, should help in translating the knowledge gained in the laboratory to the bedside.

References

[1]   Cameron AJ, Shaw JE, Zimmet PZ. The metabolic syndrome: prevalence in worldwide populations. *Endocrinol. Metab. Clin. North. Am.* 2004;33:351-375.

[2]   Reaven GM. Insulin resistance, cardiovascular disease, and the metabolic syndrome: how well do the emperor's clothes fit? *Diabetes Care* 2004;27:1011-1012.

[3]   Ross R: Atherosclerosis: an inflammatory disease. *N. Engl. J. Med.* 1999;340:115–126.

[4]   Wannamethee SG, Lowe GD, Shaper AG, Rumley A, Lennon L, Whiner PH, Insulin resistance, haemostatic and inflammatory markers and coronary heart disease risk factors in type 2 diabetic men with and without coronary heart disease. *Diabetologia.* 2004;47(9):1557-1565.

[5]   Sjoholm A, Nystrom T. Endothelial inflammation in insulin resistance. *Lancet* 2005;365(9459):610-612.

[6]   Ceriello A, Motz E. Is oxidative stress the pathogenic mechanism underlying insulin resistance, diabetes, and cardiovascular disease? The common soil hypothesis revisited. *Arterioscler. Thromb. Vasc. Biol.* 2004;24:816-823.

[7]   Hansson JK. Inflammation, atherosclerosis, and coronary artery disease. *N. Engl. J. Med.* 2005;352:1685-1695.

[8]   Black PH. The inflammatory response is an integral part of the stress response: Implications for atherosclerosis, insulin resistance, type II diabetes and metabolic syndrome X. *Brain. Behav. Immun.* 2003 Oct;17(5):350-64. Review.

[9]   Shinozaki K, Kashiwagi A, Masada M, Okamura T. Molecular mechanisms of impaired endothelial function associated with insulin resistance. *Curr. Drug. Targets Cardiovasc. Haematol. Disord.* 2004;4:1-11.

[10]   Fernandez-Real JM, Ricart W. Insulin resistance and chronic cardiovascular inflammatory syndrome. *Endocr. Rev.* 2003;24(3):278-301.

[11]   Reaven GM, Laws A. Insulin resistance, compensatory hyperinsulinaemia, and coronary heart disease. *Diabetologia.* 1994;37(9):948-52.

[12]   Expert Panel on Detection, Evaluation, and Treatment of High Blood Cholesterol in Adults: Executive Summary of the Third Report of the National Cholesterol Education Program (NCEP) Expert Panel on Detection, Evaluation, and Treatment of High Blood Cholesterol in Adults (Adult Treatment Panel III). *JAMA,* 2001;285:2486-2497.

[13]   International Diabetes Federation: The IDF consensus worldwide definition of the metabolic syndrome. IDF Executive Office, Brussels, Belgium. *www.idf.org.*

[14]   Clinical guidelines on the Identification, Evaluation, and Treatment of Overweight and Obesity in Adults – The Evidence Report, National Institutes of Health. *Obes. Res.* 1998;6(suppl 2):51S-209S.

[15]   Sung RY, Tong PC, YU CW, et al. High prevalence of insulin reistance and metabolic syndrome in overweight/obese preadolescent Homg Kong Chinese children aged 9-12 years. *Diabetes Care* 2003;26:250-151.

[16]   Chan JC, Cheung JC, Stehouwer CD, Emeis JJ, Tong PC, Ko GT, Yudkin JS. The central roles of obesity-associated dyslipidaemia, endothelial activation and cytokines in the Metabolic Syndrome--an analysis by structural equation modelling. *Int. J. Obes. Relat. Metab. Disord.* 2002;26(7):994-1008.

[17] Tracy RP. Inflammation, the metabolic syndrome and cardiovascular risk. *Int. J. Clin. Pract. Suppl.* 2003;134:10-17.

[18] Danesh J, Wheeler JG, Hirschfield GM, et al. C-reactive protein and other markers of inflammation in the prediction of coronary artery disease. *N. Engl. J. Med.* 2004;350:1387-1397.

[19] Wannamethee SG, Lowe GD, Shaper AG, Rumley A, Lennon L, Whiner PH, Insulin resistance, haemostatic and inflammatory markers and coronary heart disease risk factors in type 2 diabetic men with and without coronary heart disease. *Diabetalogia* 2004;47(9):1557-1565.

[20] Muntner P, He J, Chen J, Fonseca V, Whelton PK. Prevalence of non-traditional cardiovascular risk factors among persons with impaired fasting glucose, impaired glucose tolerance, diabetes, and the metabolic syndrome: analysis of the Third National Health and Nutrition Examination Survey (NHANES III). *Ann. Epidemiol.* 2004;14(9):686-695.

[21] Hsueh WA, Quinones MJ. Role of endothelial dysfunction in insulin resistance. *Am. J. Cardiol.* 2003;92:10J-17J.

[22] Pearson TA, Mensah GA, Alexander RW, et al. Markers of inflammation and cardiovascular disease: application to clinical and public health practice: a statement for healthcare professionals from the Centers for Disease Control and Prevention and the American Heart Association. *Circulation* 2003;107:499-511.

[23] Ridker PM, Cushman M, Stampfer MJ, Tracy RP, Hennekens CH. Inflammation, aspirin, and the risk of cardiovascular disease in apparently healthy men. *N. Engl. J. Med.* 1997;336:973-979. (*Erratum, N. Engl. J. Med.* 1997;337:356).

[24] Ridker PM, Rifai N, Rose L, Buring JE, Cook NR. Comparison of C-reactive protein and low-density lipoprotein cholesterol levels in the prediction of first cardiovascular events. *N. Engl. J. Med.* 2002;347-1557-1565.

[25] Bruno G, Cavallo-Perin P, Bargero G, et al. Hyperfibrinogenemia and metabolic syndrome in type 2 diabetes: a population-based study. *Diabetes. Metab. Res. Rev.* 2001;17(2): 124-130.

[26] Carr ME. Diabetes mellitus: a hypercoagulable state. *J. Diabetes. Complications.* 2001;15(1):44-54.

[27] Stehouwer CDA, Gall M, Twisk JWR, Knudsen E, Emeis JJ, Parving H. Increased urinary albumin excretion, endothelial dysfunction, and chronic low-grade inflammation in type 2 diabetes. Progressive, interrelated, and independently associated with risk of death. *Diabetes* 2002;51:1157-1165.

[28] Duncan BB, Schmidt MI, Pankow JI, et al. Low-grade systemic inflammation and the development of type 2 diabetes. The Atherosclerosis Risk in Communities study. *Diabetes* 2003;52:1799-1805.

[29] Freeman DJ, Norrie J, Caslake MJ, et al. C-reactive protein is an independent predictor of risk for the development of diabetes in the West of Scotland Coronary Prevention Study. *Diabetes* 2002;51:1596-1600.

[30] Asakawa H, Tokunaga K, Kawakami F. Elevation of fibrinogen and thrombin-antithrombin III complex levels of type 2 diabetes patients with retinopathy and nephropathy. *J. Diabetes. Complications.* 2000;14(3):121-126.

[31] Saraheimo M, Teppo AM, Forsblom C, Fagerudd J, Groop PH. Diabetic nephropathy is associated with low-grade inflammation in type 1 diabetic patients. *Diabetalogia* 2003;46(10):1402-1407.

[32] Tall AR. C-reactive protein reassessed. *N Engl J Med* 2004;350:1450-1452.

[33] Mosca L. C-reactive protein – to screen or not to screen? *N. Engl. J. Med.* 2002;347:1615-1617.

[34] Hackam DG, Anand SS. Emerging risk factors for atherosclerotic vascular disease: a critical review of the evidence. *JAMA* 2003;290(7):932-940.

[35] Streja D, Cressey P, Rabkin SW. Associations between inflammatory markers, traditional risk factors, and complications in patients with type 2 diabetes mellitus. *J. Diabetes Complications* 2003;17(3):120-127.

[36] Bhatt DL, Topol EJ. Need to test the inflammation hypothesis. *Circulation* 2002;106:136-140.

[37] Ceriello A, Motz E. Is oxidative stress the pathogenic mechanism underlying insulin resistance, diabetes, and cardiovascular disease? The common soil hypothesis revisited. *Arterioscler. Thromb. Vasc. Biol.* 2004;24:816-823.

[38] Ridker PM, Buring JE, Cook NR, Rifai N. C-reactive protein, the metabolic syndrome, and risk of incident cardiovascular events: an 8-year follow-up of 14,719 initially healthy American women. *Circulation* 2003;107:391–397.

[39] Pradhan AD, Cook NR, Buring JE, Manson JE, Ridker PM. C-reactive protein is independently associated with fasting insulin in nondiabetic women. *Arterioscler. Thromb. Vasc. Biol.* 2003;23:650–655.

[40] Rutter MK, Meigs JB, Sullivan LM, D'Agostino RB Sr, Wilson PW. C-reactive protein, the metabolic syndrome, and prediction of cardiovascular events in the Framingham Offspring Study. *Circulation* 2004;110:380–385.

[41] Yudkin JS, Stehouwer CD, Emeis JJ, Coppack SW. C-reactive protein in healthy subjects: associations with obesity, insulin resistance, and endothelial dysfunction: a potential role for cytokines originating from adipose tissue? *Arterioscler. Thromb. Vasc. Biol.* 1999;19:972–978.

[42] Festa A, D'Agostino R Jr, Howard G, Mykkanen L, Tracy RP, Haffner SM. Chronic subclinical inflammation as part of the insulin resistance syndrome: the Insulin Resistance Atherosclerosis Study (IRAS). *Circulation* 102:42–47, 2000

[43] Ridker PM, Wilson PW, Grundy SM. Should C-reactive protein be added to metabolic syndrome and to assessment of global cardiovascular risk? *Circulation* 2004;109:2818–2825.

[44] Isomaa B, Almgren P, Tuomi T, Forsen B, Lahti K, Nissen M, Taskinen MR, Groop L. Cardiovascular morbidity and mortality associated with the metabolic syndrome. *Diabetes Care* 2001;24:683-689.

[45] Alexander CM, Landsman PB, Teutsch SM, Haffner SM, Third National Health and Nutrition Examination Survey (NHANES III), National Cholesterol Education Program (NCEP): NCEP-defined metabolic syndrome, diabetes, and prevalence of coronary heart disease among NHANES III participants age 50 years and older. *Diabetes* 2003;52:1210-1214.

[46] Freeman DJ, Norrie J, Caslake MJ, et al. C-reactive protein is an independent predictor of risk for the development of diabetes in the West of Scotland Coronary Prevention Study. *Diabetes* 2002;51:1596-1600.

[47] Pradhan A, Manson J, Rifai N, Buring J, Ridker P. C-reactive protein, interleukin 6, and risk of developing type 2 diabetes mellitus. *JAMA* 2001;286:3327-334.

[48] Hackam DG, Anand SS. Emerging risk factors for atherosclerotic vascular disease: a critical review of the evidence. *JAMA* 2003;290(7):932-940.

[49] Danesh J, Wheeler JG, Hirschfield GM, Eda S, Eiriksdottir G, Rumley A, Lowe GD, Pepys MB, Gudnason V: C-reactive protein and other circulating markers of inflammation in the prediction of coronary heart disease. *N. Engl. J. Med.* 2004;350: 1387-1397.

[50] Ridker PM, Rifai N, Rose L, Buring JE, Cook NR: Comparison of C-reactive protein and low-density lipoprotein cholesterol levels in the prediction of first cardiovascular events. *N. Engl. J. Med.* 2002;347: 1557-1565.

[51] McLaughlin T, Abbasi F, Lamendola C, Liang L, Reaven G, Schaaf P, Reaven P: Differentiation between obesity and insulin resistance in the association with C-reactive protein. *Circulation* 2002;106:2908-2912.

[52] Danesh J, Collins R, Appleby P, Peto R. Association of fibrinogen, C-reactive protein, albumin, or leukocyte count with coronary heart disease: meta-analyses of prospective studies. *JAMA* 1998;279:1477–1482.

[53] Ridker PM, Hennekens CH, Buring JE, Rifai N. C-reactive protein and other markers of inflammation in the prediction of cardiovascular disease in women. *N. Engl. J. Med.* 2000;342:836–843.

[54] Ridker PM. Clinical applications of C-reactive protein for cardiovascular disease detection and prevention. *Circulation* 2003;107:363–369.

[55] Ridker PM, Cannon CP, Morrow D, Rifai N, Rose LM, McCabe CH, Pfeffer MA, Braunwald E. C-reactive protein levels and outcomes after statin therapy: Pravastatin or Atorvastatin Evaluation and Infection Therapy-Thrombolysis in Myocardial Infarction 22 (PROVE IT-TIMI 22). *N. Engl. J. Med.* 2005;352:20–28.

[56] Ridker PM, Buring JE, Cook NR, Rifai N. C-reactive protein, the metabolic syndrome, and risk of incident cardiovascular events: an 8-year follow-up of 14,719 initially healthy American women. *Circulation* 2003;107:391–397.

[57] Pradhan AD, Cook NR, Buring JE, Manson JE, Ridker PM. C-reactive protein is independently associated with fasting insulin in nondiabetic women. *Arterioscler. Thromb. Vasc. Biol.* 2003;23:650–655.

[58] Yudkin JS, Stehouwer CD, Emeis JJ, Coppack SW. C-reactive protein in healthy subjects: associations with obesity, insulin resistance, and endothelial dysfunction: a potential role for cytokines originating from adipose tissue? *Arterioscler. Thromb. Vasc Biol.* 1999;19:972–978.

[59] McLaughlin T, Abbasi F, Lamendola C, Liang L, Reaven G, Schaaf P, Reaven P. Differentiation between obesity and insulin resistance in the association with C-reactive protein. *Circulation* 2002;106:2908–2912.

[60] Festa A, D'Agostino R Jr, Howard G, Mykkanen L, Tracy RP, Haffner SM. Chronic subclinical inflammation as part of the insulin resistance syndrome: the Insulin Resistance Atherosclerosis Study (IRAS). *Circulation* 2000;102:42–47.

[61] Sattar N, Gaw A, Scherbakova O, Ford I, O'Reilly DS, Haffner SM, Isles C, Macfarlane PW, Packard CJ, Cobbe SM, Shepherd J. Metabolic syndrome with and without C-reactive protein as a predictor of coronary heart disease and diabetes in the West of Scotland Coronary Prevention Study. *Circulation* 2003;108:414–419.

[62] Rutter MK, Meigs JB, Sullivan LM, D'Agostino RB Sr, Wilson PW. C-reactive protein, the metabolic syndrome, and prediction of cardiovascular events in the Framingham Offspring Study. *Circulation* 2004;110:380–385.

[63] Reilly MP, Wolfe ML, Rhodes T, Girman C, Mehta N, Rader DJ. Measures of insulin resistance add incremental value to the clinical diagnosis of metabolic syndrome in association with coronary atherosclerosis. *Circulation* 2004;110:803–809.

[64] Trujillo ME, Scherer PE. Adiponectin – journey from an adipocyte secretory protein to biomarker of the metabolic syndrome. *J. Intern. Med*.2005;257(2):167-175.

[65] Chandran M, Phillips SA, Ciaraldi T, Henry RR. Adiponectin: more than just another fat cell hormone? *Diabetes Care* 2003;26:2442–2450.

[66] Weyer C, Funahashi T, Tanaka S, Hotta K, Matsuzawa Y, Pratley RE, Tataranni PA. Hypoadiponectinemia in obesity and type 2 diabetes: close association with insulin resistance and hyperinsulinemia. *J. Clin. Endocrinol. Metab*.2001;86:1930–1935.

[67] Matsubara M, Maruoka S, Katayose S. Decreased plasma adiponectin concentrations in women with dyslipidemia. *J. Clin. Endocrinol. Metab.* 2002;87:2764–2769.

[68] Kazumi T, Kawaguchi A, Sakai K, Hirano T, Yoshino G. Young men with high-normal blood pressure have lower serum adiponectin, smaller LDL size, and higher elevated heart rate than those with optimal blood pressure. *Diabetes Care* 2002;25:971–976.

[69] Kumada M, Kihara S, Sumitsuji S, Kawamoto T, Matsumoto S, Ouchi N, Arita Y, Okamoto Y, Shimomura I, Hiraoka H, Nakamura T, Funahashi T, Matsuzawa Y, Osaka CAD Study Group. Association of hypoadiponectinemia with coronary artery disease in men. *Arterioscler. Thromb. Vasc. Biol.* 2003;23:85–89.

[70] Kojima S, Funahashi T, Sakamoto T, Miyamoto S, Soejima H, Hokamaki J, Kajiwara I, Sugiyama S, Yoshimura M, Fujimoto K, Miyao Y, Suefuji H, Kitagawa A, Ouchi N, Kihara S, Matsuzawa Y, Ogawa H. The variation of plasma concentrations of a novel, adipocyte derived protein, adiponectin, in patients with acute myocardial infarction. *Heart* 2003;89:667–672.

[71] Zoccali C, Mallamaci F, Tripepi G, Benedetto FA, Cutrupi S, Parlongo S, Malatino LS, Bonanno G, Seminara G, Rapisarda F, Fatuzzo P, Buemi M, Nicocia G, Tanaka S, Ouchi N, Kihara S, Funahashi T, Matsuzawa Y. Adiponectin, metabolic risk factors, and cardiovascular events among patients with end-stage renal disease. *J. Am. Soc. Nephrol.* 2002;13:134–141.

[72] Pischon T, Girman CJ, Hotamisligil GS, Rifai N, Hu FB, Rimm EB. Plasma adiponectin levels and risk of myocardial infarction in men. *JAMA* 2004;291:1730–1737.

[73] Kershaw EE, Flier JS: Adipose tissue as an endocrine organ. *J. Clin. Endocrinol. Metab.* 2004;89:2548–2556.

[74] Yudkin JS, Stehouwer CD, Emeis JJ, Coppack SW. C-reactive protein in healthy subjects: associations with obesity, insulin resistance, and endothelial dysfunction: a potential role for cytokines originating from adipose tissue? *Arterioscler. Thromb. Vasc Biol* 1999;19:972–978.

[75] McCarty MF. Interleukin-6 as a central mediator of cardiovascular risk associated with chronic inflammation, smoking, diabetes, and visceral obesity: down-regulation with essential fatty acids, ethanol, and pentoxifylline. *Med. Hypotheses.* 1999;52(5):465-477.

[76] Fasshauer M, Paschke R. Regulation of adipocytokines and insulin resistance. *Diabetologia* 2003;46(12):1594-1603.

[77] Vozarova B, Weyer C, Hanson K, et al. Circulating interleukin-6in relation to adiposity, insulin action, and insulin secretion. *Obes. Res.* 2001:9:414-417.

[78] Bastard JP, Jardel C, Bruckert E, Blondy P, Capeau J, Laville M, Vidal H, Hainque B. Elevated levels of interleukin 6 are reduced in serum and subcutaneous adipose tissue of obese women after weight loss. *J. Clin. Endocrinol. Metab.* 2000;85:3338-3342.

[79] Hotamisligil GS. Adipose expression of tumor necrosis factor: direct role in obesity-linked insulin resistance. *Science* 1993:259:87-91.

[80] Kern PA, Saghizadeh M, Ong JM, Bosch RJ, Deem R, Simsolo RB. The expression of tumor necrosis factor in human adipose tissue: regulation by obesity, weight loss, and relationship to lipoprotein lipase. *J. Clin. Invest.* 1995:95:2111-2119.

[81] Otero M, Lego R, Lago F, el al. Leptin, from fat to inflammation: old questions and new insights. *FEBS Lett* 2005;579(2):295-301.

[82] Unger RH. Longevity, lipotoxicity, and leptin: the adipocyte defense against feasting and famine. *Biochimie* 2005;87(1):57-64.

[83] Franks PW, Brage S, Luan J, Ekelund U, Rahman M, Farooqi IS, et al. Leptin predicts a worsening of the features of the metabolic syndrome independently of obesity. *Obes. Res.* 2005;13(8):1476-1484.

[84] Ridker PM, Rifai N, Pfeifer MA, Sacks FM, Moye LA, Goldman S, et al. Inflammation, pravastatin, and the risk of coronary events after myocardial infarction in patients with average cholesterol levels. *Circulation* 1998;98(9)839-844.

[85] Ernst E, Resch KL: Fibrinogen as a cardiovascular risk factor: a meta-analysis and review of the literature. *Ann. Intern. Med.* 18:956–963, 1993

[86] Imperatore G, Riccardi G, Iovine C, Rivellese AA, Vaccaro O: Plasma fibrinogen: a new factor of the metabolic syndrome: a population-based study. *Diabetes Care* 21:649–654, 1998

[87] Schram MT, Stehouver CD. Endothelial dysfunction, cellular adhesion molecules and the metabolic syndrome. *Horm. Metab. Res.* 2005;37(suppl 1):49-55.

[88] Potter van Loon BJ, Kluft C, Radder JK, Blankenstein MA, Meinders AE: The cardiovascular risk factor plasminogen activator inhibitor type 1 is related to insulin resistance. *Metabolism* 42:945–949, 1993

[89] Festa A, D'Agostino R Jr, Mykkanen L, Tracy RP, Zaccaro DJ, Hales CN, Haffner SM: Relative contribution of insulin and its precursors to fibrinogen and PAI-1 in a large population with different states of glucose tolerance: the Insulin Resistance Atherosclerosis Study (IRAS). *Arterioscler. Thromb. Vasc. Biol.* 19:562–568, 1999

[90] Dandona P, Aljada A, Chaudhuri A, Mohanty P, Garg R. Metabolic syndrome: a comprehensive perspective based on interactions between obesity, diabetes, and inflammation. *Circulation* 2005;111(11):1448-1454.

[91] Conlan MG, Folsom AR, Finch A, Davis CE, Sorlie P, Marcucci G, et al. Associations of factor VIII and von Willibrand factor with age, race, sex, and risk factors for atherosclerosis: the atherosclerosis risk in communities (ARIC) study. *Thromb. Haemost.* 1993;70:380-385.

[92] Janand-Delenne B, Chagnaud C, Raccah D, Alessi MC, Juhan-Vague I, Vague P. Visceral fat as a main determinant of plasminogen activator inhibitor 1 level in women. *Int. J. Obes. Relat. Metab. Disord.* 1998;22:312-317.

[93] Sakkinen PA, Wahl P, Cushman M, Lweis MR, Tracy RP. Clustering of procoagulation, inflammation, and fibrinolysis variables with metabolic factors in insulin resistance syndrome. *Am. J. Epidemiol.* 2000;152:897-907.

[94] Juhan-Vague I, Pyke SD, Alessi MC, Jespersen J, Haverkate F, Thompson SG. Fibrinolytic factors and the risk of myocardial infarctionor sudden death in patients with angina pectoris: ECAT study group. European concerted action on thrombosis and disabilities. *Circulation* 1996;94:2057-2063.

[95] Cook DG, Mendall MA, Whincup PH, Carey IM, Ballam L, Morris JE, Miller GJ, Strachan DP: C-reactive protein concentration in children: relationship to adiposity and other cardiovascular risk factors. *Atherosclerosis* 2000;149:139–150.

[96] Visser M, Bouter LM, McQuillan GM, Wener MH, Harris TB: Low-grade systemic inflammation in overweight children. *Pediatrics* 200;107:E13.

[97] Wu DM, Chu NF, Shen MH, Chang JB: Plasma C-reactive protein levels and their relationship to anthropometric and lipid characteristics among children. *J. Clin. Epidemiol.* 2003;56:94–100.

[98] Vikram NK, Misra A, Dwivedi M, Sharma R, Pandey RM, Luthra K, Chatterjee A, Dhingra V, Jailkhani BL, Talwar KK, Guleria R: Correlations of C-reactive protein levels with anthropometric profile, percentage of body fat and lipids in healthy adolescents and young adults in urban North India. *Atherosclerosis* 2003;168:305–313.

[99] Must A, Jacques PF, Dallal GE, Bajema CJ, Dietz WH: Long-term morbidity and mortality of overweight adolescents: a follow-up of the Harvard Growth Study of 1922 to 1935. *N. Engl. J. Med.* 1992;327:1350–1355.

[100] Gungor N, Thompson T, Sutton-Tyrrell K, Janosky J, Arslanian S. Early signs of cardiovascular disease in youth with obesity and type 2 diabetes. *Diabetes Care* 2005;28:1219-1221.

[101] Sorrentino MJ. Implications of the metabolic syndrome: the new epidemic. *Am. J. Cardiol.* 2005;96(4A):3E-7E.

[102] Pritchett AM, Foreyt JP, Mann DL. Treatment of the metabolic syndrome: the impact of lifestyle modification. *Curr. Atheroscler. Rep.* 2005;7(2):95-102.

[103] Esposito K, Marfella R, Ciotola M, Di Palo C, Giugliano F, Giugliano G, D'Armiento M, D'Andrea F, Giugliano D. Effect of a mediterranean-style diet on endothelial dysfunction and markers of vascular inflammation in the metabolic syndrome: a randomized trial. *JAMA* 2004;292(12):1440.

[104] Riserus U, Basu S, Jovinge S, Fredrikson GN, Arnlov J, Vessby B. Supplementation with conjugated linoleic acid causes isomer-dependent oxidative stress and elevated C-reactive protein: a potential link to fatty acid-induced insulin resistance. *Circulation* 2002;106(15):1925-1929.

[105] Luyckx FH, Lefebvre PJ, Scheen AJ. Non-alcoholic steatohepatitis: association with obesity and insulin resistance, and influence of weight loss. *Diabetes Metab.* 2000;26(2):98-106.

[106] Pitsavos C, Panagiotakos DB, Chrysohoou C, Kavouras S, Stefanadis C. The associations between physical activity, inflammation, and coagulation markers, in people with metabolic syndrome: the ATTICA study. *Eur. J. Cardiovasc. Prev. Rehabil.* 2005;12(2):151-158.

[107] Troseid M, Lappegard KT, Claudi T, Damas JK, Morkrid L, Brendberg R, Mollnes TE. Exercise reduces plasma levels of the chemokines MCP-1 and IL-8 in subjects with the metabolic syndrome. *Eur. Heart. J.* 2004;25(4):349-355.

[108] Bray GA, Champagne CM. Obesity and the Metabolic Syndrome: implications for dietetics practitioners. *J. Am. Diet. Assoc.* 2004;104(1):86-89.

[109] Ishizaka N, Ishizaka Y, Toda E, Hashimoto H, Nagai R, Yamakado M. Association between cigarette smoking, metabolic syndrome, and carotid arteriosclerosis in Japanese individuals. *Atherosclerosis.* 2005;181(2):381-388.

[110] Chu JW, Abbasi F, Lamendola C, McLaughlin T, Reaven GM, Tsao PS. Effect of rosiglitazone treatment on circulating vascular and inflammatory markers in insulin-resistant subjects. *Diab. Vasc. Dis. Res.* 2005;2(1):37-41.

[111] Arner P. The adipocyte in insulin reistance: key molecules and the impact of the thiazolidinediones. *TRENDS in Endocrinol. Metab.* 2003;14(3):137-145.

[112] Iushibashi M, Egashira K, Hiasa K, Inoue S, Ni W, Zhao Q, et al. Antiinflammatory and antiarteriosclerotic effects of pioglitazone. *Hypertension* 2002;40:687-693.

[113] Scandinavian Simvastatin Survival Study Group. Randomised trial of cholesterol lowering in 4444 patients with coronary heart disease: the Scandinavian simvastatin survival study (4S). *Lancet* 1994;344:1383-9.

[114] Kinjo K, Sato H, Sakata Y, et al. Relation of C-reactive protein and one-year survival after acute myocardial infarction with versus without statin therapy. *Am J Cardiol* 2005;96(5):617-621.

[115] Elrod JW, Lefer DJ. The effects of statins on endothelium, inflammation, and cardioprotection. *Drugs News Perspect* 2005;18(4):229-236.

[116] Jialal I, Stein D, Balis D, Grundy SM, Adams-Huet B, Devaraj S: Effects of hydroxymethyl glutaryl coenzyme A reductase inhibitor therapy on high sensitive C-reactive protein levels. *Circulation* 2001;103:1933-1935.

[117] Maki KC. Fibrates for treatment of the metabolic syndrome. *Curr. Atheroscler. Rep.* 2004 J;6(1):45-51.

[118] Dagenais NJ, Jamali F. Protective effects of angiotensin II interruption: evidence for antiinflammatory actions. *Pharmacotherapy* 2005;25(9):1213-1229.

[119] Sierra C, de la Sierra A. Antihypertensive, cardiovascular, and pleiotropic effects of angiotensin-receptor blockers. *Curr. Opin. Nephrol. Hypertens.* 2005;14(5):435-441.

[120] American College of Endocrinology (ACE) Position Statement on the Insulin Resistance Syndrome. *Endocr. Pract.* 2003;9(No. 3):236-252.

[121] van Oostrom AJ, van Wijk J, Cabezas MC. Lipaemia, inflammation and atherosclerosis: novel opportunities in the understanding and treatment of atherosclerosis. *Drugs* 2004;64 Suppl 2:19-41.

[122] Garg R, Tripathy D, Dandona P. Insulin resistance as a proinflammatory state: mechanisms, mediators, and therapeutic interventions. *Curr. Drug. Targets.* 2003;4(6):487-492.

In: Progress in Metabolic Syndrome Research
Editor: George T. Ulrig, pp. 111-130

ISBN 1-60021-179-8
© 2006 Nova Science Publishers, Inc.

Chapter V

Genetic Polymorphisms Linked to Metabolic Syndrome

Ana Z. Fernandez[1],* and Mercedes T. Fernandes-Mestre[2]

[1]Lab. Trombosis Eperimental, Centro de Biofisica y Bioquimica, Instituto Venezolano de Investigaciones Cientificas IVIC. Caracas 1020A Venezuela.

[2]Lab. Fisiopatologia, Centro de Medicina Experimental, IVIC. Caracas 1020A Venezuela.

Abstract

Metabolic syndrome (MS) comprises a range of alterations associated with glucose and lipid homeostasis disturbances, all conditions which are strongly influenced by each individual's genetic and environmental factors. In addition to Insulin resistance, abdominal obesity and dyslipidemia, arterial blood pressure, pro-inflammatory and pro-thrombotic states have also been included as major components of MS. This multifaceted composition implies that many metabolic pathways could be genetically altered. In humans, there has been described a number of single nucleotide polymorphisms (SNP) and deletion/insertion polymorphisms in different genes linked to glucose metabolism (Insulin receptor *IR*, protein tyrosine phosphatase 1β PTPβ*)*, blood pressure (beta-adrenergic receptors *BAR*, renin-angiotensin system RAS, Nitric Oxide Sintase NOS*)*, lipoprotein variations (Cholesteryl ester transfer protein *CETP*, Apolipoproteins AI, C-III, and E), lower Body Mass Index (Leptin, Peroxisome proliferator-activated receptors *PPAR*, uncoupling protein *UCP*), some inflammatory components (C Reactive protein *CRP)* and the hemostatic system (plasminogen-activator inhibitor *PAI-1)*, among others. The purpose of this review is to compile recent evidence that could link genetic variations of different genes with the phenotypic features of MS.

* Correspondence concerning this article should be addressed to Ana Z. Fernandez1, PhSc. Lab. Trombosis Eperimental, Centro de Biofisica y Bioquimica, Instituto Venezolano de Investigaciones Cientificas IVIC. Km11 Carretera Panamericana, postal code 21827 Caracas 1020A Venezuela. Email: azitaf@ivic.ve.

Keywords: Insulin resistance, dyslipidemia, polymorphisms, multifactorial

Introduction

In spite of the relatively recent boom on metabolic syndrome (MS), this is not a new finding (Eckel et al 2005). Initially known as Insulin Resistance Syndrome and/or Syndrome X, MS has been defined in clinical practical terms by having three of the following conditions (Roberts 2004): (1) abdominal obesity (increased waist circumference above 102cm in men and 88cm in women); (2) serum triglycerides levels higher than 150mg/dl (> 3.82 mmol/L); (3) high density lipoprotein (HDL) levels below 40 mg/dl (<1.03 mmol/L) in men and 50 mg/dl (<1. 30 mmol/L) in women; (4) high systemic arterial blood pressure (≥ 130/ ≥ 85 mmHg); and (5) fasting blood glucose level above 110 mg/dl. This classical definition of MS comprises four essential elements: glucose intolerance, obesity, hypertension and dyslipidaemia (Fig 1). However, several disturbances on both the immune (proinflammatory) and the hemostatic (prothrombotic) system have also gained attention (Grundy, 2003).

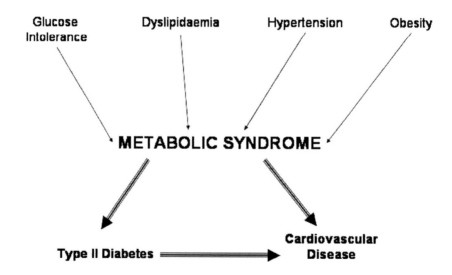

Figure 1. Four essentials elements of Metabolic Syndrome and its harmful consequences

MS is the harmful onset for cardiovascular disease and type II diabetes (Reaven 1988; Liese et al. 1998). It has been established that individual with MS have three-fold relative risk of undergoing cardiovascular disease (Haffner et al 2003), and a higher predictive value of being affected by type II diabetes (Grundy et al. 2004). World prevalence has been *in crescendo,* being the Hispanic ethnics the most susceptible (Haffner et al 2003).

The most common type of human genetic variation is the single nucleotide polymorphism (SNP), a position at which two alternative bases occur with appreciable frequency (>1%) in the human population. SNPs can serve as genetic markers for identifying disease genes by linkage studies in families, linkage disequilibrium in isolated populations, association analysis of patients and controls, and loss-of-heterozygosity in tumors (Wang et al., 1998). Insertion-deletion polymorphism is also found, but at a relative low frequency. Obviously, there are too many known and unknown metabolic pathways involved, affected or interconnected in MS, and each one of these is a potential target for present and further genetic research.

Genetic Polymorphisms of Insulin Signal Transduction Pathway

Insulin, the hormone secreted by the pancreatic β-cells, is probably one of the most important signal regulators in mammals. In fact, insulin-regulated metabolic pathways have been studied with a special and particular interest, since disturbances in its regulation could trigger the development of insulin resistance, followed by MS and finally, diabetes.

First of all, a primary metabolic effect of insulin is to stimulate the uptake of circulating glucose into muscle and adipose tissue, a critical step in glucose metabolism, through the insulin-regulatable glucose transporter isotype 4 (Glut4) (Fig.2). In a sequence of processes not fully dilucidated until now, insulin stimulates glucose uptake by eliciting the translocation of intracellular Glut4-containing vesicles to the cell surface (Ross et al. 2004). In addition to stimulating glucose uptake into skeletal muscle and adipose tissue, insulin also inhibits the hepatic output of glucose by inhibiting the transcription of key gluconeogenic enzymes and inducing the transcription of key glycolytic enzymes.

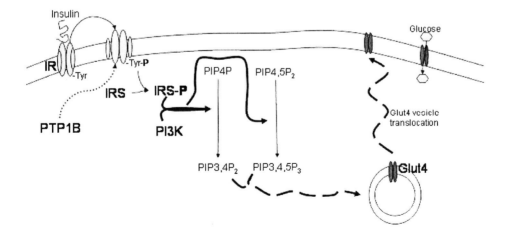

Figure 2. Binding of insulin to insulin receptor IR results in the releasing of Tyrosine kinase activity on insulin receptor Substrates (IRS). IRS associate with class 1A phosphatidylinositol 3' kinase (PI3K). This interaction activates de catalytic subunit of PI3K to phosphorylate the 3' position of phosphatidylinositol 4-phosphate (PIP4P) and phosphatidylinositol 4,5-biphosphate (PIP4,5P$_2$) to form phosphatidylinositol 3,4-biphospahate (PIP3, 4P2) and phosphatidylinositol 3,4,5-triphosphate (PIP3,4,5P$_3$), respectively. Activation of PI3K has been found critical in mediating Glut4 vesicle translocation and glucose transport in response to insulin (Ross t al 2004). Regulation of IR tyrosine kinase activity is achieved by Protein Tyrosine Phosphatase 1B (PTP1B).

Insulin binds to its receptor (Insulin Receptor IR), a member of the receptor tyrosine kinase family, which in turn propagates insulin signaling via tyrosine phosphorylation of substrate proteins. Insulin receptor is a heterotetramer, two allosteric inhibitory alpha subunits and two catalytic beta subunits. Binding of insulin to IR results in the autophosphorylation on tyrosine 1146,1150 and 1151 of alpha regulatory subunit and releasing of tyrosine kinase activity (White and Kahn 1994) on at least nine substrate proteins (Ross et al 2004). Tyrosine-phosphorylated Insulin receptor Substrates (IRS) proteins associate with class 1A phosphatidylinositol 3' kinase (PI3K). This interaction activates de catalytic subunit of PI3K to phosphorylate the 3' position of phosphatidylinositol 4-phosphate and phosphatidylinositol 4,5-biphosphate to form phosphatidylinositol 3,4-biphosphate and phosphatidylinositol 3,4,5-triphosphate, respectively. Activation of PI3K has been found critical in mediating Glut4 vesicle translocation and glucose transport in response to insulin (Ross et al 2004).

Insulin Receptor IR

Some evidences have been found that correlate IR gene variants with disturbances in blood pressure. Thus, an increase in the prevalence of the IR gene RsaI restriction fragment-length polymorphism (RFLP) major allele (7.0kb) has been reported in Australian white hypertensive when compared with normotensive subjects (Morris, 1997). Aditionally, the P1 allele and homozygous genotype frequencies of an IR gene PstI RFLP were higher in hypertensive Polish subjects when compared with normotensive subjects (Pissarska, 1996). The silent mutation in exon 8 of the IR gene in an A-to-G transition at nucleotide 6224, introducing an NsiI restriction site, where the N1 allele lacks the restriction site, has also been associated to hypertension (Thomas et al., 2000). This IR gene *Nsi*I RFLP was found to be weakly associated with diastolic blood pressure in Hong Kong Chinese subjects with varying aspects of the MS, but there was no association between the NsiI RFLP and insulin resistance, suggesting that insulin resistance may not be the mechanism through which the IR receptor could influence diastolic blood pressure (Thomas et al. 2000).

Protein Tyrosine Phosphatase 1B

It has been found that the IR-dependent tyrosine kinase activity could be regulated by the Protein Tyrosine Phosphatase 1β (PTP1β) (Kennedy et al. 2000). Disruption of the PTP1 β activity caused enhanced insulin sensitivity and resistance to weight gain in double knockout mice (Elchebly et al 1999). These findings correlated with an increment in tyrosine phosphorylation of the IR and IRS.

PTP1β is a ubiquitously expressed protein implicated in negative regulation of insulin signaling, by dephosphorylating the phosphotyrosine residues of the IR. The 10 exons of *PTPN1*, the gene for PTP-1β, span >74kb of chromosome 20q13.13. Polymorphisms of *PTPN1* have been associated with type 2 diabetes (Mok Et al., 2002; Echwald et al., 2002), plasma lipids levels, total plasma cholesterol, body mass index and hypertension (Olivier et al., 2004). This last study support the idea that PTP-1β affects plasma lipid levels, and may lead to obesity and hypertension. It has been identified at least 35 SNP across of the genomic region containing *PTPN1* associated with quantitative measures of glucose homeostasis (Palmer et al 2004). Aditionally, it was detected by Spencer-Jones et al. in a study on normal female population (n=2,777; mean age, 47.4 ± 12.5 years) that *PTPN1* protective haplotype was associated with high insulin sensitivity index, low triglyceride level and low systolic blood pressure (Spencer-Jones et al. 2005).

Genetic Polymorphims of Lipoprotein-Linked Proteins

Lipoproteins are dinamic multicomponent complexes of proteins (apolipoproteins) and lipids (cholesterol and cholesterol esters, phospholipids and triacylglycerols), which interact with different enzymes and lipid transfer proteins, molding their composition, density and diameter throughout their time life. Five classes of plasma lipoproteins exist; they are classified according to their density: chylomicrons (d<0.95 gr/mL), very low density lipoprotein (VLDL, d= 0.95-1.006 gr/mL), intermediate density lipoprotein (IDL, d=1.006-1.019 gr/mL), low density lipoprotein (LDL, d= 1.019-1.063 gr/mL) and high density lipoprotein (HDL, d= 1.063-1.210 gr/mL). The central function of lipoproteins is the transport of cholesterol and other lipids, function that is achieved by three interconnected and interdependent pathways: 1) the transport of dietary or exogenous fats; 2) the transport of hepatic or endogenous lipids; and 3) reverse cholesterol transport (Kwiterovich 2000).

Briefly, dietary fat is secreted from intestinal cells on chylomicrons in a process that requires apolipoprotein B-48. Meanwhile, triglyceride-rich VLDL is synthesized and secreted from the liver in a process that requires apolipoprotein B-100. The triglycerides in the core of the chylomicrons and VLDL are hydrolyzed into free fatty acids and glycerol by lipoprotein lipase with apolipoprotein C-II as cofactor, producing smaller chylomicron remnants and VLDL remnants. Chylomicrons remnants are removed by apoE/apoB receptor on liver, while VLDL remnants are further transformated into IDL. Some of the IDL particles are removed through the interaction of apolipoprotein E with the LDL receptor on the surface of the liver, or the triglycerides in IDL can be hydrolyzed by hepatic lipase to produce LDL. LDL is normally uptaken by the interaction of apolipoprotein B-100 with the LDL receptor (Kwiterovich 2000). At the same time, enterocytes and hepatocytes produce lipid-poor Apolipoprotein A-I-containing particles, which interact with peripheral cells and acquire phospholipids and free cholesterol through ATP-binding cassette protein A1 (ABCA1) (Chan et al., 2004). Phospholipid transfer protein (PLTP) also facilitates the transfer of phospholipids from cellular membranes and lipoprotein surfaces to form pre-beta-HDL. Once associated with nascent HDL, free cholesterol is esterified by the enzyme Lecithin: cholesterol acyltransferase (LCAT). Cholesteryl esters can also be selectively transferred to apoB-containing lipoprotein in exchange for tryglicerides through the action of Cholesteryl ester transfer Protein (CETP). The maturation to higher cholesterol-rich HDL particles is due to continuous acquisition of free cholesterol and its subsequent esterification (Chan et al., 2004).

An already mentioned feature closely linked with MS is dyslipidemia, a simplified description for the so called, "atherogenic lipoprotein triad" characterized by accumulation of triacylglycerol-rich lipoproteins and small dense LDL with depressed HDL-cholesterol levels (Chan et al., 2004). Numerous clinical and epidemiological studies have demonstrated that plasma concentrations of HDL-C and apoA-I are inversely correlated with coronary heart disease (CHD) (Boden 2000; Wang and Briggs, 2004).

Different polymorphisms of genes encoding proteins involved in lipid metabolism have been associated with variations in lipoprotein levels. Major mutations have been described in genes for LDL receptor (LDLR), apolipoprotein B (ApoB) and LDL-adaptor protein (Falchi et al. 2004). The most commonly reported gene defects in patients with a low HDL-cholesterol involve the ABCA1, apoA-I and LCAT. The magnitude of the effect of each of these polymorphisms is generally small but, when combined, may lead to major changes. A brief description and genetic variants of some lipoprotein-related proteins follows.

Apolipoproteins A

Apolipoprotein A-I is the most important apolipoprotein in HDL, representing almost 70% of HDL protein. ApoA-I participates by two mechanisms in the reverse transport of cholesterol: 1) by stimulating cholesterol efflux from cells via the ABCA1 transporter protein associated with the cellular membranes (Chan et al., 2004), and 2) by acting as cofactor for LCAT (Breslow, 1985; Chroni et al., 2005). The apoAI gene is 1863bp in length and has been mapped to chromosome 11 in humans (Breslow, 1985). Mutations of ApoAI have been correlated with normal or reduced HDL levels and have been described at least 50 variants until now. ApoAI$_{Milano}$ (Arg173Cys) and ApoAI$_{Paris}$ (Arg151Cys) are examples of natural variants of ApoAI that manifest HDL deficiencies, but paradoxically carriers of these mutations seem to be protected against cardiovascular disease (Bielicki and Oda, 2002). Other mutations result from substitutions of aminoacids (Pro143Arg in ApoAI$_{Giessen}$, Asp103Asn in ApoAI$_{Munster3A}$, Pro4Arg in ApoAI$_{Munster3B}$, Pro3His in ApoAI$_{Munster3C}$) and stop transcription. Recently Dastani et al. described a novel ApoA-I mutation (ApoA-IE136X) in a French Canadian population with low HDL-Cholesterol (HDL-C) levels, where glutamic acid at position 136 of ApoA-I is substituted by a stop signal, producing a truncated mutant (Dastani et al. 2005). Interestingly, in three probands for ApoA-IE136X and 14 heterozygous carriers with the very low levels of HDL (0.51 ±0.16 mmol/L), 13 out of 17 had a Body Mass Index (BMI) higher than 25 kg/m^2 and 3 subjects had hipertriglyceridemia. Although Dastani et al. pointed out that no probands had diabetes, they did no mention about diabetes or insulin resistance in their carrier relatives and also, in spite the authors indicated that blood pressure was taking to each individual, no data were reported concerning this parameter. Moreover, some of the subjects in this study were found to show premature coronary artery disease (Dastani et al. 2005).

Many genetic investigations have shown that MspI polymorphisms in ApoA-I gene are correlated with changes of HDL-C and ApoA-I. A common adenine for guanine substitution located -78bp upstream from the ApoA-I gene transcription start site (MspI 1) and a cytosine to thymine transition at +83bp of the ApoA-I gene (MspI 2) can destroy the MspI restriction sites (Jia et al. 2005). In a recent research in China, where 307 subjects were studied, Jia et al found that G/A and A/A polymorphisms in MspI 1 site were correlated with higher triglyceride levels, apoC-II, apoC-III, apoA-I contents of preβ-HDL and HDL3 and TG/HDL-C ratio compared to G/G polymorphism both in females and males groups, while the C/T and C/C polymorphisms in MspI 2 site did not show significant differences in plasma lipids, lipoproteins and apolipoproteins (Jia et al., 2005).

Apolipoprotein A-II is the second most abundant protein in HDL comprising approximately 20 % of HDL protein (Breslow, 1985). *In vitro* apoA-II has been shown to displace apoA-I from HDL particles as well as both activate hepatic lipase and inhibit LCAT (Breslow, 1985). The Apo A-II gene has been mapped to human chromosome 1 (1q21-q23), and a few mutations on apoA-II gene has been identified. A polymorphism of the apolipoprotein AII gene was investigated using genomic hybridisation analysis. The two common alleles at this locus were defined by MspI restriction fragments of 3.0 kilobase pairs (M3.0) and 3.7 kilobase pairs (M3.7) respectively. The M3.7 allele was significantly more common (P less than 0.02) in Caucasian subjects who were normolipemic (34%, 20/59) than in those who were hypertriglyceridaemic (16%, 16/98). Serum triglycerides levels were measured in 126 Caucasian subjects with different combinations of disease-associated alleles at the ApoAII and ApoCIII gene loci. Mean serum triglycerides levels were found to be significantly higher (P less than 0.05) in subjects with disease-associated alleles of both the ApoCIII and ApoAII genes, compared with subjects with a disease-associated allele of one or neither locus (Ferns et al 1986).

Apolipoprotein B

This is the major protein constituent of LDL but is also found in Chylomicrons, VLDL and IDL. Human ApoB is a glycoprotein which occurs in two forms, designated B-100 (4536 amino acids) and B-48 (2152 amino acids), the first one has a hepatic origin and is the protein component in LDL, while the second one is sinthetized in the intestine as component of chylomicrons. The high plasmatic level of apoB-100 and LDL-C has been correlated with cardiovascular disease (Hurt-Camejo and Camejo, 1999).The ApoB gene has been mapped to human chromosome 2 (2p24-p23) and it produces both apoB-100 and ApoB-48 by a unique mRNA editing process (Whitfield et al 2004). Mutations in the *APOB* gene causing the production of a truncated molecule can cause familial hypobetalipoproteinemia and hypocholesterolemia, whereas defects in the carboxy terminus of the LDL-receptor-binding domain of apoB cause a form of hypercholesterolemia (Whitfield et al 2004). Numerous polymorphisms have been described in this gene. The XbaI polymorphism is one of the most studied and, although this mutation does not modify the primary structure, it has been demonstrated trat the presence of the X+ allele (sequence recognized by the XbaI restriction enzyme) is correlated with high cholesterol and TG levels in plasma (Ordovás 1999).

Apolipoprotein Cs

The genes coding for human apoC-I and human apoC-II are members of a 48-kb gene cluster on chromosome 19, that also includes the *APOE* and pseudo-*APOC1'* genes (Jong et al. 1999). It has been reported that the human *APOC1* gene is located either 4.3 or 5.3 kb downstream from the *APOE* gene in the same transcriptional orientation. The *APOC1* gene is aproximately 4.7 kb and is primarily expressed in the liver, but lower amounts are also found to be expressed in the lung, skin, testes, and spleen. *APOC2* spans a region of 3.4 kb and is primarily expressed in the liver and intestine. The human *APOC3* gene is located in a gene cluster together with the *APOA1* and *APOA4* genes on the long arm of chromosome 11 and is approximately 3.1 kb, mostly expressed in liver and intestine (Jong et al.1999).

ApoC-I in HDL may modulate LCAT activity. One population-based, genetic association study has reported an *Hpa*I RFLP in the *APOC1* promoter, located at a site 317 bp 59 from the apoC1 transcription initiation site. Under certain conditions, the *Hpa*I promoter variant causes overexpression of *APOC1,* which may contribute to the development of hyperlipidemia

As already mentioned, ApoC-II is the cofactor for lipoprotein lipase. Genetic defects in the structure or production of human apoC-II are linked to high circulating levels of triglycerides and are phenotypically indistinguishable from patients with Lipoprotein Lipase deficiency (Jong et al. 1999). Sequence analysis of the *APOC2* gene in families with familial hyperchylomicronemia has revealed a variety of molecular defects in this particular gene. In 7 families (Nijmegen, Paris, Barcelona, Japan, Venezuela, Padova, and Bari), a single base change resulted in the introduction of a premature stop that led to the synthesis of truncated forms of apoC-II that were either not secreted or rapidly cleared from the circulation (Jong et al. 1999). A donor splice-site mutation in the first base of the second intron of the *APOC2* gene was found in a Hamburg family and in a neonatal Japanese patient (*APOC2*Hamburg and *APOC2*Tokyo, respectively). This mutation caused abnormal splicing of APOC2 mRNA and was associated with low levels of apoC-II in plasma. In addition, a variety of single–amino acid substitutions in the *APOC2* gene has been described that either resulted in the inability to initiate apoC-II synthesis or in the production of nonfunctional apoC2 (Jong et al.1999). For 2 *APOC2* variants (*APOC2*SanFrancisco and the *APOC2* Lys193Thr mutation), a direct relationship between this mutant form of apoC2 and lipoprotein abnormalities could not be established.

ApoC-III has been implicated as Lipoprotein lipase inhibitor. Several lines of evidence have implicated apoC-III as possibly contributing to the development of hypertriglyceridemia. A positive correlation has been observed between plasma apoC-III levels and elevated levels of plasma VLDL-TGs. However, structural mutations in the human *APOC3* gene fail to clearly show an association between the mutation and an altered lipid/lipoprotein metabolism. Variable degree of sialylation on ApoC-III seems to reflect little or no influence on lipoprotein metabolism, since carriers of mutations at the glycosylation site were normolipidemic. The *APOC3* Lys583Glu mutation was associated with low plasma apoC-III concentrations and atypically large HDL (Von Eckardstein et al 1991). The Asp453Asn variant was found in a Turkish patient who underwent coronary bypass surgery but failed to show a clear association between the mutation and an abnormal lipoprotein metabolism. The *APOC3* Gln383Lys mutation was observed in a boy of Mexican origin, and family studies in 16 individuals who were heterozygous for this *APOC3* mutation revealed mildly elevated levels of plasma TGs in these subjects. Several studies have also reported a complete apoC3 deficiency in families with an increased prevalence of premature coronary heart disease. However, in all cases, apoC3 deficiency was associated with an apoAI deficiency, making it difficult to estimate the exact contribution of the lack of apoC3 to changes in lipoprotein levels.

In addition to the genetic mutations described above, several restriction fragment length polymorphisms (RFLPs) in or around the human *APOC* genes have been identified that are associated with lipoprotein disorders or altered plasma lipid concentrations in humans. These are an *Sst*I RFLP in the noncoding region of exon 4 of the *APOC3* gene, a C11003T polymorphism in exon 3 of the *APOC3* gene and RFLPs within the *APOA1/C3/A4* gene cluster such as *Xmn*I and *Pst*I. It has been demonstrated that a minor allele (*S2*) of an *Sst*I RFLP in the *APOC3* gene is associated with hypertriglyceridemia in several distinct populations. Other RFLPs within the *APOA1/C3/A4* gene cluster such as *Xmn*I and *Pst*I have also been reported to be associated with hypertriglyceridemia or coronary artery disease.

Apolipoprotein E

Apolipoprotein E comprises about 10-20% of VLDL protein and 1-2% of HDL protein, and its main function is to serve as ligand for apoB/E receptor present on hepatic as well as extrahepatic tissues (Breslow, 1985). Apo E gene is about 3.7kb in length, and contains four exons and three introns. The gene has been mapped to human chromosome 19 (Breslow, 1985). Three common polymorphisms exist through a C>T transition leading to variations in the amino acids (Cys>Arg) at 112 and 158 positions, resulting in three major alleles, named ε2, ε3 and ε4, with relative frequencies of 0.1, 0.8 and 0.15, respectively (Vincent et al. 2002). The protein product of apoE- ε 2 gene binds poorly to the remnant receptor, leading to accumulation of TG-rich lipoprotein in the circulation, while the apoE- ε 4 gene product has high affinity for its receptor, which increases TG-rich lipoprotein uptake by the liver, thus inducing a down-regulation of the apoB/E receptor, with subsequent reduction of LDL uptake and increasing LDL accumulation (Vincent et al. 2002).

Cholesteryl Ester Transfer Protein

Cholesteryl ester transfer protein (CETP) is important for HDL metabolism because this lipid transfer protein enables the transfer of cholestery ester from HDL toward TG-rich lipoproteins and LDL. Evidence is accumulating that common polymorphisms in the CETP gene influence HDL-C levels. Also, mutations in CETP may have different effects in men and women, since HDL-C levels in women are ussually higher compared to those in men.

The TaqIB polymorphism in intron 1 of the *CETP* has been most widely studied, although it is closely linked to the -629 C>A promoter polymorphism in the same gene (Borggreve et al. 2005). In homozygous people for the TaqIB CETP polymorphism restriction locus B1B1, a high CETP activity associated with low plasma HDL-C levels can be measured. The lowest CETP activity combined with high HDL-C levels, meaning a protective cardiovascular effect has, on the other hand, been described for homozygous subjects for the B2 allele, denoting the absence of the restriction locus (Weitgasser et al 2004). Furthermore, it has been shown that the effect of statin treatment in patients with significant coronary disease is enhanced in the presence of a B2 allele (Carlquist et al 2003).

The -629 C>A *CETP* promoter variant does not alter the molecular structure of this lipid transfer protein but affects the amount of active CETP in serum, where this genotype is correlated with higher levels of HDL-C and ApoA-I (Borggreve et al 2005). However, it was found in a population-based study that TG levels could influence negatively the effect of this promoter polymorphism on HDL-C, which gives to this CETP gene-TG interaction an interpretation of genetic effects on the HDL phenotype and could be of help to predict the effect of TG-lowering treatment on raising HDL-C (Borggreve et al. 2005).

On the other hand, it has been shown for a white female population that elevated HDL-C caused by the Ile405Val mutation in the CET gene is a risk factor for ischemic heart disease (Agerholm-Larse et al. 2000).

ATP-Binding Cassette transporter 1 (ABCA1)

ABCA1 is a transporter protein that mediates the transfer of cholesterol and phospholipids from peripheral cells to lipid-poor apoA-I. The *ABCA1* gene is contained within a 149-kb chromosomal locus on human chromosome 9 and comprises 50 exons encoding a 250-kDa protein. Disruption in ABCA1 function due to mutations in the *ABCA1* gene causes Tangier Disease and familial hypoalphalipoproteinemia, which are characterized by low to absent HDL levels and an increased deposition of cholesteryl esters in several tissues and cells (Wang and Briggs, 2004), while the overexpression of this gene seems to confer protection against atherosclerosis (Singaraja et al. 2002).

Other ABC transporters may also play roles in lipoprotein homeostasis. The transporters ABCG5 and ABCG8 have been implicated in efflux of dietary sterols from intestinal cells back into the gut lumen and from the liver to the bile duct (Wang and Briggs, 2004). In hmans, mutations in the ABCG5 (G5) and ABCG8 (G8) genes result in pathologically high intestinal absorption of cholesterol and phytosterols. In a study in Finland, Gylling et al found that in a moderately hypercholesterolemic population, subjects with the lowest tertile of serum cholestanol-to-cholesterol ratio, a surrogate marker of low cholesterol absorption efficiency, had characteristic of the MS (Gylling et al. 2004); aditionally, they found that the Asp19His polymorphism of the *G8* gene was strongly associated with cholesterol absorption in men and the Gln604Glu polymorphism of the *G5* gene was associated with fasting insulin (Gylling et al 2004). However, there is not a straight explanation for linking how genes that regulate cholesterol absorption could regulate insulin action or interact with gender.

Genetic Polymorphisms of Blood Pressure Regulators

The pathogenesis of hypertension is still not fully understood, however several studies have reported that an alteration in nitric oxide (NO) metabolism may be an important factor in its development (Forte et al, 1997; Huang et al 1995). Likewise, different investigations have demonstrated that mutations affecting the endothelial NO (eNOS) gene may compromise endothelial NO synthesis and predispose individuals with the mutant allele to the development of hypertension.

Nitric oxide (NO), a potent vasodilator produced by endothelial cells, plays an important role in the regulation of blood pressure and regional blood flow, and also inhibits platelet aggregation and leukocyte adhesion to vascular endothelium (Takaota 2004). Moreover, NO seems to modulate glucose metabolism and insulin secretion, which suggests an aditional role for NO in the insulin-resistance and diabetes evolution (Pieper, 1999; Piatti et al., 2000; Zavaroni et al., 2000). NO is sinthesized from L-Arginine by the action of NO sinthetases (NOS). Constitutively expressed endothelial NOS (eNOS) produce low concentrations of NO, necessary for a good endothelial function and integrity (Albrecht et al 2003), however various genetic polymorphisms of the eNOS gene have been reported as susceptibility genes in myocardial infarction (Shismasaki et al 1998) hypertension (Miyamoto et al., 1998; Shoji et al., 2000) and coronary artery spasm (Yoshimura 1998; Nakajama et al. 1999). For example, hypertensive patients have impaired NO-mediated dilation of the small resistance vessels, which leads to an elevation in blood pressure. Nakajama et al. demonstrated that the variant T-786→C in the eNOS 5' flanking region gene, principally the C/C genotype decrease promoter activity (Nakajama et al., 1999). Similarly, another study reported that the -786C allele decreased eNOS mRNA levels and serum nitrate and nitrite (Miyamoto et al, 2000). Hyndman et al (2002) reported that the -786C allele was over-represented in hypertensive patients and that subjects with the C/C genotype had significantly higher systolic blood pressures and therefore were more likely to be hypertensive, suggesting that this genotype is a significant factor to increase the risk of essential hypertension (Hyndman et al., 2002). Most recently, the 1132T>C polymorphism, within the promoter of the NOS3 gene, was reported to be associated with metabolic syndrome in hypertensive patients (Fernandez et al., 2004). Also, the G to T conversion at nucleotide 894 in the eNOS gene, which introduces an aspartic acid in place of glutamic acid (Glu298Asp) has been suggested to play a role in the development of hypertension. Veldman et al reported that the eNOS Glu298Asp polymorphism is associated with reduced basal NO production and might therefore have functional implications in the development of atherosclerosis or hypertension (Veldman et al., 2002).

Another genetic polymorphism associated with components of the metabolic syndrome is the type II SH2 domain-containing inositol 5-phosphatase (*INNPPL1* or SHIP2). *INNPPL1* is a negative regulator of insulin and *Innppl1* inactivation in mice results in increased insulin sensitivity (Clement et al., 2001). Kaisaki et al observed significant associations of SNPs and haplotypes of *INNPPL1* with hypertension as well as with other components of the MS (Kaisaki et al., 2004). This group reported the strongest association between hypertensive and three *INNPPL1* SNPs, rs2276047, snp8 and rs9886. Also, the haplotype I-A-G (snp8-

rs2276047- rs9886) was most frequent in diabetic patients with hypertension compared with those without hypertension, concluding that *INNPPL1* variants may confer susceptibility to disease and/or to sub phenotypes involved in the MS in diabetic patients.

As hypertension has been related to sodium intake, and many patients with essential hypertension are overweight and have the MS, studies on microsatellite markers close to the thiazide-sensitive Na-Cl co-transporter on chromosome 16 and a quantitative trait locus for abdominal obesity-metabolic syndrome on chromosome 17 have been recently started (Cheung et al., 2005). Significant differences were observed in the distribution of D17S1303 among hypertensive individuals and normal controls, while the number of GATA repeats correlated inversely with diastolic blood pressure. Nine GATA repeats in D17S1303 were associated with hypertension and 14 GATA repeats with normotension, suggesting an association of D17S1303 microsatellite marker with essential hypertension.

The association between the C825T polymorphism in the GNB3 gene, which encodes the beta 3 subunit of heterotrimeric G proteins and hypertension, has been reported. Individuals with the 825T allele have an increased risk of hypertension combined with features of MS, such as dyslipidemia, hypercholesterolemia, insulin resistance and obesity (Siffert 2005). Moreover, 825T allele carriers respond with a stronger decrease in blood pressure to therapy with thiazide diuretic and clonidine (Sartori et al., 2004), however further studies are needed to use this polymorphism in clinical practice and for individualized treatment regimens (Siffert, 2005).

Endogenous catecholamines are important modulators of adipose tissue lipolysis, glucose homeostasis and vascular tone (Insel 2000) controlling several pathways of the MS. In humans, tissue catecholamines exert their effects through different β-adrenergic receptors (BAR), clustered in three subtypes (BAR1, BAR2 and BAR3). Two SNPs at nucleotides 46 and 79 of the BAR2 gene result in the substitution of an amino acid in the extracellular domain of the receptor: Gly16Arg and Gln27Glu (Green et al 1994). These polymorphisms have been associated with hypertension and other components of the MS, such as obesity, insulin resistance and dyslipidemia. Dallongeville et al studied the relation between BAR2 polymorphisms (Gly16Arg and Gln27Glu) and each component of the MS individually (Dalongeville et al., 2003). The results showed a gene-dose association between BAR2 SNPs and low HDL cholesterol, glucose intolerance and high blood pressure supporting the concept that polymorphisms on a unique gene with ubiquitous effects on metabolic pathways may increase the susceptibility to MS.

The renin-angiotensin system (RAS) plays a key role in the regulation of blood pressure. Renin converts angiotensinogen to angiotensin 1, which in turn is converted to the vasoconstrictor angiotensin 2 by angiotensin 1 converting enzyme (ACE). Inhibition of the RAS by ACE-inhibitors lowers blood pressure, a widely used therapy for hypertension. It has been reported in Caucasian subjects that levels of ACE are correlated with the insertion/deletion genotype (I/D), with highest levels of ACE in those DD individuals compared to II individual (Rigat et al. 1990). Furthermore, this polymorphism has been associated to myocardio infarction (Tiret et al. 1993), and in type II diabetics, it is associated to hypertension (Wierzbiciki et al. 1995; Pujia et al. 1994) and macrovascular disease (Ruiz et al. 1994). However, several studies of the influence of ACE I/D polymorphism on macrovascular and/or microvascular disease show variable results (Nagi et al. 1998). Further studies of the I/D polymorphism could be of particular interest since it has been suggest that plasmatic levels of ACE are associated with characteristic features of MS.

Genetic Polymorphisms Related to Abdominal Obesity

The function of adipose tissue is to provide enery to the organism during periods when energy from exogenous nutrients is not available. This can be divided into two phases, one between meals, for example during sleep, and the other during periods when supply of energy from nutrients is not available, followed by starvation for days or longer periods. Nowadays, the situation is that starvation periods are extremely uncommon and the need for this reserve function of adipose tissue hardly exists any longer, so that the adipose tissue capacity to store fat is now excessive (Björntorp 1999). Even more, adipose tissue is an endocrine organ that may affect the function of other organs in the whole body by secreting a variety of adipocytokines (Matsuzawa 2005). For many years efforts to identify candidate genes for obesity have been concentrated on adipose tissue.

The standard unit of measure to determine obesity is body mass index (BMI), which is weight divided by the square of one's height. People with a BMI of 25-30 kg/m^2 are considered overweight, while those above 30 are obese. Other measurement is the waist-to-hip ratio, which is an estimated of the abdominal fat distribution. In fact, it has been consistently shown in a large number of studies, that excess fat assembled in central abdominal depots is a powerful risk factor for the development of cardiovascular disease, type II diabetes, stroke and their metabolic and hemodynamic consequences (Björntorp 1999).

Obesity, like other conditions associated to MS, is a multifactorial condition, where environmental factors related to a sedentary lifestyle and unlimited access to food apply constant pressure in subjects with a genetic predisposition to gain weight. The fact that genetic defects can result in human obesity has been recently established with the identification of the genetic defects responsible for diferent monogenic forms of human obesity: the leptin, leptin receptor, pro-opiomelanocortin (POMC), pro-hormone convertase-1 (PC1) and melanocortin-4 receptor (MC4R) genes. The common forms of obesity are, however, polygenic (Boutin and Froguel, 2001). Leptin, which is secreted by the adipocytes in proportion to their fat content, circulates and binds the long form of the leptin receptor in the hypothalamus. POMC gene expression is increased by leptin action, which leads to the production of alpha-melanocyte-stimulating hormone (a-MSH), which reduces food intake when it binds to the brain-specific MC4 receptor.

In a family-based study designed to assess the role of leptin in association with BMI, 29SNPs spanning 240kb across the Leptin region (7q31.3) were genotyped (Yiang et al. 2004). Those results showed a strong association of a number of common variants and haplotypes in the 5' region of leptin with BMI adjusted for age and sex, which may be useful for identifying those subjects who may have a leptin deficiency and a predisposition to obesity derived from altered regulatory transcriptional elements (Yiang et al., 2004).

The Isoleucine (I) for Valine (V) polymorphism is the most common MC4R variant. In a meta-analysis led by Geller et al., it was found a negative association (odd ratio of 0.69; 95% CI 0.50 to 0.96, P =0.03) between the I103 allele and obesity (Geller et al. 2004).

On the other hand, the regulation of thermogenesis by the sympathetic nervous system is mediated by beta-adrenergic receptors. In humans, BAR3 is modestly expressed in fat and the adipocytes lining the gastrointestinal tract. A Trp64Arg mutation located in the first transmembrane domain of the receptor was identifed in obese Pima Indians and French and Finnish subjects (Clement et al. 1995; Widen et al., 1995).

Importantly, in mature brown adipocyte cells, BAR3 stimulates uncoupling protein-1 (UCP1) via a cAMP metabolic pathway. UCPs are inner mitochondrial membrane transporters that dissipate the proton gradient, releasing stored energy in the form of heat. An A to G variation in UCP1 was associated with a gain of fat mass in a Quebec family study. Additional effects of the G allele of the -3826 variant of UCP1 with the Trp64Arg mutation of the BAR3 gene were shown on weight gain in a morbid obese French population. Moreover, polymorphisms in other members of the uncoupling gene family, UCP2 and UCP3, were associated with body mass index in Pima Indians. Variations in the BAR3 and UCP genes are probably not sufficient on their own to induce obesity (Boutin and Froguel, 2001). In addition, their function is still being debated, and recent data from UCP2 knockout mice have shown no effect on body weight. In contrast, there is now evidence that UCP2 is a potent inhibitor of insulin secretion, these UCP2 knockout mice exhibiting hyperinsulinaemia. All these uncertainties illustrate the complexity of the candidate gene approach, especially when gene function is not understood (Boutin and Froguel, 2001).

Other Factors Potentially Involved in Metabolic Syndrome

C-Reactive Protein

Low –grade systemic inflammation seems to play a role in the pathobiology of various components of MS. C-reactive protein (CRP) was initially defined as a protein up-regulated as part of the acute response in humans, that binds to the polysaccharide of *Streptococcus pneumoniae* (Carlson et al. 2005). It has been suggested that increased serum CRP, which is synthesized primarily in the liver in response to interleukin-6 and other cytokines, may not only be a sensitive marker of low level inflammation but may directly enhance inflammation, through its involvement in binding to complement C1q and in activated endothelial cells (Burke et al. 2002; Jialal et al. 2004).

Elevated human serum CRP has been positively correlated to the number of atherosclerotic plaques and histologic staining for CRP in fatal lesions from autopsy samples (Burke et al. 2002). In the Women's Health Study, it was found a positive association between increasing levels of CRP and the risk of developing hypertension, with a relative risk in women with CRP levels higher than 3mg/L of 2.11 (95% CI, 1.97-2.26; Sesso et al 2003); this finding suggests that inflammation may be an important mechanism through with the hypertension develops (Sesso et al 2003).

The gene of CRP has been mapped to chromosome 1. Several polymorphisms in the CRP gene region were identified by direct resequencing of 47 individual from the Coronary Artery Risk Development in Young Adults (CARDIA) study, and then seven tagSNPs representative of all common patterns in each ethnicity were selected for genotyping in a larger panel of clinically phenotyped samples (Carlson et al. 2005). These seven tagSNPs defined eight common haplotypes. Haplotype 1(H1) (tagged by SNP2667) was associated with significantly reduced CRP levels relative to H2, and H6 (tagged by SNP790) was associated with the highest CRP levels relative to all other haplotypes (Carlson et al. 2005).

Plasminogen Activator Inhibitor-type 1

Being the hemostasia a quite complex system, their involvement in the initial steps of MS is scarcely known. However, obesity, plasma triglycerides, renin-angiotensin system as well as insulin resistance have been consistently correlated to Plasminogen Activator Inhibitor-type1 (PAI-1), the main fast-acting inhibitor of fibrinolysis activation, which plays an important role in vascular disease prevention by removing thrombi from the vascular system (Francis 2002). Plasmin, the active component of fibrinolysis, breaks down fibrin into its degradation products. Plasminogen and tissue-type plasminogen activator (t-PA) bind to the surface of fibrin where t-PA cleaves inactive plasminogen into active plasmin. T-PA is inhibited by PAI-1, which inactivates t-PA by forming an irreversible 1: 1 complex (Hoekstra et al, 2004).

PAI-1 is produced by different cell types, including endothelial cells, hepatocytes, and adipocytes. The 4G/5G polymorphism is a common single base pair insertion/deletion polymorphism in the promoter region of the PAI-1 gene that affects gene transcription. The 4G-allele has a sequence of four guanosines. The 5G-allele has a fifth guanosine inserted, which creates an additional binding site for an inhibitor, resulting in an attenuated response to transcription factors. The 4G/4G-genotype has been associated with higher PAI-1 levels compared to the 5G/5G-genotype (Eriksson et al., 1995). *In vitro* studies in human endothelial cells showed that the HindIII-polymorphism in the 3'-untranslated region of the PAI-1 gene affects PAI-1 transcription in response to insulin and lipoproteins. The 1/1-genotype showed the strongest response in PAI-1 after stimulation with insulin, and the 2/2 genotype after triggering with either VLDL or Lp(a).

Peroxisome Proliferator-Activated Receptors

Peroxisome Proliferator-activated Receptors (PPAR) constitute a subfamily of the the nuclear receptor superfamily, which act as ligand-activated transcription factor after heterodimerization with the retinoic X receptor, recognizing PPAR response elements (PPRE) in the promoter region of target genes (Chinetti et al 2000). PPAR could also repress the transcription of certain genes activated by the proinflammatory transcription factors NFkB, AP-1 and STAT-1, through the binding and sequestration of their corresponding co-factors (Chinetti et al. 2000). Three PPAR forms have been described so far: PPARα

(NR1C2), PPARγ (NR1C3) and PPARδ/β (known also as NUC1, FAAR and NR1C2); their activation is closely linked with genes involved in glucose and lipid metabolism (Fernández 2004).

The first PPARα and γ agonists were discovered before their beneficial hypolipidemic and hypoglycemic effects could be explained at the molecular level. PPAR γ agonists, such as thiazolidinediones (pioglitazone, rosiglitazone), induce significant reductions in plasma glucose and insulin; with regard to PPARα agonists, fibrates (clofibrate, gemfibrozil) are the drugs of choice for treatment of hypertrigliceridemia and other primary dyslipidemias.

Several polymorphisms have been identified in the human PPARγ gene. The most common polymorphism consists of an Alanine (A) for Proline (P) substitution at codon 12 in the PPARG2 gene (Deeb et al. 1998). The association between the *PPARG2* P12A polymorphism and risk of Coronary Heart Disease in women (Nurses' Health Study [NHS]) and men (Health Professionals Follow-up Study [HPFS]) was assessed in two nested case control studies, showing no significant differences between A12 carriers and non carriers (Pischon et al. 2005).

Conclusion

MS seems to be a partially unfold fan, in which every portion has very complicated drawings. Moreover, the task to find out the genetic make-up that can explain or even link every component in MS is hardly achieved, since every one of these components are strongly influenced by environmental and their own genetic factors. However, it is evident that exist a close interrelationship among all the components of MS, e.g., insulin resitance is linked with blood pressure, obesity is linked to dyslipidemia, inflammation is linked to obesity, and so on. It is not unthinkable that sooner than later a genetic profile for MS will be established, and this would be a useful tool in diagnosis and prevention, not only for MS, but also for the two biggest health problems, type 2 dibetes and cardiovascular diseases.

References

Albrecht et al, 2003

Agerholm-Larsen B, Nordestgaard BG, Steffensen R, Jensen G, Tybjaerg-HansenA. Elevated HDL cholesterol is a risk factor for ischemic heart disease in white women when caused by a mutation in the cholesteryl ester transfer protein gene. *Circulation* 2000;101:1907–1912.

Bielicki, J.K., Oda, M.N. Apolipoprotein A-Imilano and Apolipoprotein A-Iparis exhibit an antioxidant activity distinct from that of wild-type Apolipoprotein A-I. *Biochemistry* 2002; 41:2089-2096

Björntorp, P.A. Overweight is risking fate. *Bailleres`s Clin.Endocrinol.Metabol.* 1999; 13:47-69

Boden, W.E. High-Density lipoprotein cholesterol as an independent risk factor in cardiovascular disease: assessing the data from Framingham to the Veterans Affairs High-Density Lipoprotein Intervention trial. *Am. J. Cardiol.* 2000; 86: 19L-22L

Breslow, J.L. Human Apolipoprotein Molecular Biology and Genetic Variation. *Ann. Rev. Biochem.* 1985; 54: 699-727

Burke, A.P., et al. Elevated C-reactive Protein values and atherosclerosis in sudden coronary death. *Circulation* 2002; 105:2019-2023

Carlquist JF, Muhlestein JB, Horne BD, Hart NI, Bair TL, Molhuizen HO, et al. The cholesteryl ester transfer protein TaqIB gene polymorphism predicts clinical benefit of statin therapy in patients with significant coronary artery disease. *Am. Heart. J.* 2003;146:1007–1014.

Carlson, C.S. et al. Polymorphisms within the C-Reactive Protein (CRP) promoter region are associated with plasma levels. *Am.. J.Hum.Genet.* 2005; 77:64-77

Chan, D.C., Barrett, P.H.R., Watts G.F. Lipoprotein transport in the metabolic syndrome: methodological aspects of stable isotope kinetic studies. *Clin. Sci.* 2004; 107: 221-232

Cheung BM, Leung RY, Man YB, Wong LY and Lau CP. Association of essential hypertension with a microsatellite marker on chromosome 17. *J. Hum. Hypertens.* 2005; 19 (5): 407-11

Clement K, Vaisse C, Manning BSJ et al. Genetic variation in the beta 3 adrenergic receptor gene and an increased capacity to gain weight in patients with morbid obesity. *New England Journal of Medicine* 1995; 333: 352-354

Clement S, Krause U, Desmedt F, Tanti J-F, Behrends J, Pesesse X, Sasaki T, Penninger J. et al. The lipid phosphatase SHIP2 controls insulin sensitivity. *Nature* 2001; 409: 92-97

Dallongeville J, Helbecque N, Cottel D., Amouyel P and Meirhaeghe. The Gly^{16}→Arg^{16} and Gln^{27}→Glu^{27} Polymorphism of β2-Adrenergic Receptor Are Associated With Metabolic Syndrome in Men. *J. Clin. Endocinol. Metab.* 2003; 88: 4862-4866

Deeb SS, Fajas L, Nemoto M, Pihlajamaki J, Mykkanen L, Kuusisto J, Laakso M, Fujimoto W, Auwerx J. A Pro12Ala substitution in PPARgamma2 associated with decreased receptor activity, lower body mass index and improved insulin sensitivity. *Nat. Genet.* 1998;20:284 –287.

Echwald, S.M., Bach, H., Vestergaard, H., Richelsen, B., Kristensen, B.P. et al.: A P387L variant in protein tyrosine phosphatase-1B (PTP-1B) is associated with type 2 diabetes and impaired serine phosphorylation of PTP-1B in vitro. *Diabetes.* 2002; 51: 1-6

Eckel, RH, Grundy, SM, Zimmet, PZ. The metabolic syndrome. *Lancet* 2005; 365:1415-1428

Eriksson P, Kallin B, van't Hooft FM, et al. Allele-specific increase in basal transcription of the plasminogen-activator inhibitor 1 gene is associated with myocardial infarction. *Proc. Natl. Acad. Sci. USA* 1995; 92: 1851-5.

Falchi et al. A genomewide search using an original pairwise sampling approach for large genealogies identifies a new locus for total and low-density lipoprotein cholesterol in two genetically differentiated isolates of Sardinia. *Am. J. Hum. Genet.* 2004; 75-1015-1031

Fernandez ML. Ruiz R, Gonzalez MA, Ramirez-Lorca R, Couto C, Ramos A, Gutierrez-Tous R, Rivera JM, Ruiz A, Real LM, Grilo A. Association of NOS3 gene with metabolic syndrome in hypertensive patients. *Thromb. Haemost.* 2004; 92:413-8

Ferns, G.A., Shelley, C.S., Stocks, J., Rees, A., Paul, H., Baralle, F., Galton, D.J. A DNA polymorphism of the apoprotein AII gene in hypertriglyceridaemia. *Hum. Genet.* 1986; 74: 302-306

Forte P, Copland M, Smith LM, Milne E, Sutherland J, Benjamin N. Basal nitric oxide synthesis in essential hypertension. *Lancet,* 1997, 349: 837-842.

Francis, C.W. Plasminogen Activator Inhibitor-1 levels and polymorphisms: Association with venous thromboembolism. *Arch.Pathol.Lab.Med.* 2002; 126:1401-1404

Geller, F., reichwald, K., Dempfle, A., et al. Melanocortin-4 Receptor Gene Variant I103 is negatively associated with obesity. *Am.J.Hum.Genet.* 2004;74: 572-581

Green SA, Turki J, Innis M, Liggett SB. Amino terminal polymorphisms of the human b2-adrenergic receptor imparts distinct agonist-promoted regulatory properties. *Biochemistry* 1994; 33:9414-9419

Grundy, S.M. Inflammation, Hypertension and the Metabolic Syndrome. *JAMA* 2003; 290: 3000-3002

Grundy S.M., Brewer B., Cleemen J.I, Smith S.C., Lenfant C.: Definition of Metabolic Syndrome: Report of the National Heart, Lung, and Blood Institute/American Heart Association Conference on scientific issues related to definition. *Circulation* 2004; 109:433-438.

Haffner S., Cassells H.B.: Metabolic Syndrome – a new risk factor of coronary heart disease? *Diab.Obes.Metabol.* 2003; 5: 359-370.

Hoekstra, T., Geleijnse,J.M., Schouten, E.G., Kluft, C. Plasminogen Activator Inhibitor-type1: Its plasma determinants and relation with cardiovascular risk. *Thromb.Haemost.* 2004; 91:861-872

Huang PL, Huang Z, Mashimo H, Bloch KD, Moskowitz MA, Bevan JA, Fishman MC. Hypertension in mice lacking the gene for endothelial nitric oxide synthase. *Nature,* 1995; 377: 239-242

Hurt-Camejo, E., Camejo, G. Mecanismos Aterogenicos de las lipoproteinas. In: *Hiperlipemias Clinica y Tratamiento.* Carmena, R., Ordovas, J.M., pp63-83. Ed. Doyma. Barcelona España.

Hyndman ME, Parsons HG, Verma S, Bridge PJ, Edworthy S, Jones C, Lonn E, Charbonneau F and Anderson TJ. The T-786→C Mutation in Endothelial Nitric Oxide Synthase Is Associated With Hypertension. *Hypertension* 2002, 39: 919-922

Insel PA. Seminars in medicine of the Beth Israel Hospital, Boston. Adrenergic receptors: evolving concepts and clinical implications. *N. Egland. J. Med* .2000; 334: 580-585

Jia, L., Bai, H., Fu, M., Xu, Y., Yang, Y., Long, S. Relationship between plasma HDL subclasses distribution and ApoA-I gene polymorphisms. *Clin.Chim.Acta* 2005; 360: 37-45

Jialal, I., Devaraj, S., Venugopal, S.K. C-Reactive Protein: Risk marker or Mediator in Atherothrombosis? *Hypertension* 2004; 44:6-11

Jong, M.C., Hofker, M.H., Havekes, L.M. Role of ApoCs in lipoprotein metabolism. *Arterioscler.Thromb.Vasc.Biol.* 1999; 19:472-484

Kaisaki P, Delépine m, Woon PY, Sebag-Montefiori L, Wilder SP, Menzel S, Vionnet N, Marion E, Riveline J-P, et al. Polymorphisms in Type II SH2 Domain-Containing

Inositol 5-Phosphatase (*INNPPL1*, SHIP2) Are Associated With Physiological Abnormalities of the Metabolic Syndrome. *Diabetes* 2004; 153: 1900-1904

Kennedy, B.P. and Ramachandran, C.: Protein tyrosine phosphatase-1B in diabetes. *Biochem. Pharmacol.* 2000; 60: 877-883

Kwiterovich, P.O. The metabolic pathways of High-Density Lipoprotein, Low-Density Lipoprotein, and triglycerides. A Current Review. *Am. J. Cardiol.* 2000; 86: 5L-10L

Liese AD, Mayer-Davis EJ, Haffner SM. Development of the multiple metabolic syndromes: an epidemiologic perspective. *Epidemiol Rev.* 1998; 20:157-172.

Matsuzawa Y. Adipocytokines and Metabolic Syndrome. *Semin.Vasc.Med.* 2005; 5:34-39

Miyamoto Y, Saito Y, Kajiyama N, Yoshimura M, Shimasaki Y, Nakayama M, Kamitami S, Harada M, Ishikawa M, Kuwahara K, Ogawa E, Hamanaka I, Takahashi N, Kaneshige T, Teraoka N, Akamizu T. et al. Endothelial nitric oxide synthase gene is positively associated with essential hypertension. *Hypertension.*1998; 32: 3-8.

Miyamoto Y, Saito Y, Nakayama M, Shimasaki Y, Yoshimura T, Yoshimura M, Harada M, Kajiyama N, et al. Replication protein A1 reduces transcriptrion of the endothelial nitric oxide synthase gene containing a T-786→C mutation associated with coronary spastic angina. *Hum. Mol. Genet.* 2000; 9:2629-2637

Mok, A., Cao, H., Zinman, B., Hanley, A.J., Harris, S.B. et al.: A single polymorphism in protein tyrosine phosphatase PTP-1B is associated with protection from diabetes or impaired glucose tolerance in Oji-Cree. *J. Clin. Endocrinol. Metab.* 2002; 87: 724-727

Morris, B.J. Insulin Receptor gene in hypertension. *Clin. Exp. Hypertens.* 1997; 19: 551-565.

Nakajama M, Yasue H, Yoshimura M, Shimasaki Y, Kugiyama K, Ogawa H, Motoyama T, Saito Y, et al. T-786→C mutation in the 5'- flanking region of the endothelial nitric oxide synthase gene is associated with coronary spasm. *Circulation.* 1999; 99: 2864-2870

Olivier, M., Hsiung, Ch. A., Chuang, L.M., Ho, L.T., Ting, Ch-T. et al.: Single nucleotide polymorphisms in protein tyrosine phosphatase 1B (PTPN1) are associated with essential hypertension and obesity. *Human Molecular Genetics.* 2004; 13(17): 1885-1892

Ordovas, J.M. Genetica de las hiperlipemias. In: *Hiperlipemias Clinica y Tratamiento.* Carmena, R., Ordovas, J.M., pp41-62. Ed. Doyma. Barcelona España.

Pischon, T., Pai, J.K., Manson, J.E., et al. Peroxisome Proliferator-Activated Receptor-γ-2 P12A Polymorphism and Risk of Coronary Heart Disease in US Men and Women. *Arterioscler. Thromb. Vasc. Biol.* 2005; 25: 1654-1658

Pissarska, M. Polymorphic variability of apolipoprotein B and insulin receptor genes in essential hypertension. *Pol. Arch. Med. Wewn.* 1996; 95:205-211

Reaven GM. Banting lecture 1988: role of insulin resistance in human disease. *Diabetes.* 1998 37: 1595-1607

Roberts, W.C.: The Metabolic Syndrome. *Am. J. Cardiol.* (2004) 93: 274

Ross, S.A., Gulve, E. A., Wang, M. Chemistry and Biochemistry of Type 2 Diabetes. *Chem. Rev.* 2004; 104: 1255-1282

Sesso, H.D., Buring, J.E., Rifai, N., Blake, G.J., Gaziano, J.M., Ridker, P.M. C-Reactive Protein and the risk of developing hypertension. *JAMA* 2003; 290: 2945-2951

Siffert W. G protein polymorphism in hypertension, atherosclerosis and diabetes. *Annu. Rev. Med.* 2005; 56:17-28

Singaraja, R.R., Fievet, C., Castro, G., et al. Increased ABCA-1 activity protects against atherosclerosis. *J.Clin.Invest.* 2002;110: 35-42

Shismasaki Y., Yasue H, Yoshimura M, Nakayama M, Kugiyama K, Ogawa H, Harada E, Masuda T, Koyama W, Saito Y, Miyamoto Y, Ogawa Y, Nakao K. Association of the missense Glu298Asp variant of the endothelial nitric oxide gene with myocardial infarction. *J. Am. Coll. Cardiol.* 1998; 31:1506-1510

Shoji M, Tsutaya S, Saito R, Takamatu H, Yasujima M. Positive association of endothelial nitric oxide synthase gene polymorphism with hypertension in northern Japan. *Life Sci.* 2000; 66: 2557-2562

Spencer-Jones, N.J., Wang, X., Snieder, H., Spector, T.D., Carter, N.D., O'Dell, S.D. Protein Tyrosine Phosphatase-1B Gene *PTPN1* Selection of Tagging Single Nucleotide Polymorphisms and Association With Body Fat, Insulin Sensitivity, and the Metabolic Syndrome in a Normal Female Population. *Diabetes* 2005, 54: 3296-3304

Startori M, Parotto E, Ceolotto G, Papparella I, Lenzini L, Calo LA, Semplicini A. [C825T polymorphism of the GNB3 gene codifying the g-protein beta-3 subunit and cardiovasvular] *Ann. Ital. Med. Int.* 2004; 19 (4):240-8

Takaota M. NOS gene polymorphism. *Nippon. Rinsho*, 2004; 62(1):103-9

Thomas, G.N., Tomlinson, B., Chan, J.C.N., Lee,Z.S.K., Cockran, C.S., Critchley, J.A.J.H. An Insulin Receptor Gene Polymorhism is Associated with Diastolic Blood Pressure in Chinese Subjects with Components of the Metabolic Syndrome. *Am. J. Hypertens.* 2000; 13: 745-752

Veldman BA, Spiering W, Doevendans PA, Vervoort G, Kroon AA, de Leeuw PW, Smits P. The Glu298Asp polymorphism of the NOS 3 gene as a determinant of the baseline production of nitric oxide. *J. Hypertens.* 2002; 20(10):2023-7.

Von Eckardstein A., Holz, H., sandKamp M., Weng W., Funke H., Assman G. Apolipoprotein C-III (Lys58->Glu). Identification of an apolipoprotein C-III variant in a family with hyperalphalipoproteinemia. *J.Clin.Invest.* 1991; 87: 1724-1731

Wang, D.G., et al. Large-scale Identification, Mapping, and Genotyping of Single-Nucleotide Polymorphism in the Human Genome. *Science* 1998; 1077-1082

Wang, M., Briggs, M.R. HDL: Themetabolism, function and Therapeutic Importance. *Chem. Rev.* 2004; 104: 119-137

Weitgasser, R., Galvan, G., Malaimare L., et al. Cholesteryl ester transfer protein TaqIB polymorphism and its relation to parameters of the insulin resistance syndrome in an Austrian Cohort. Biomed. *Pharmacother.*2004; 58: 619-627

Widen E, Lehto M, Kanninen T et al. Association of a polymorphism in the beta3-adrenergic receptor gene with features of the insulin resistance syndrome in Finns. *New England Journal of Medicine* 1995; 333: 348-352

Whitfield, A.J., Barrett, P.H.R., van Bockxmeer, F.M., Burnett, J.R. Lipid disorders and mutations in the APOB gene. *Clin. Chem.* 2004; 50:1725-1732

Yoshimura M, Yasue H, Nakayama M, Shimasaki Y, Sumida H, Sugiyama S, Kugiyama K. et al. A missense Glu298Asp variant in the endothelial nitric oxide gene is associated with coronary spasm in Japanese. *Hum. Genet.* 1998; 103: 65-69

Index

N

O

P

S

T

U

V

W

Y